T0234546

OTHER FAST FACTS BOOKS

Fast Facts on **ADOLESCENT HEALTH FOR NURSING AND HEALTH PROFESSIONALS**: A Care Guide *(Herrman)*

Fast Facts for the **ANTEPARTUM AND POSTPARTUM NURSE**: A Nursing Orientation and Care Guide *(Davidson)*

Fast Facts Workbook for **CARDIAC DYSRHYTHMIAS AND 12-LEAD EKGs** *(Desmarais)*

Fast Facts for the **CARDIAC SURGERY NURSE**: Caring for Cardiac Surgery Patients, Third Edition *(Hodge)*

Fast Facts for **CAREER SUCCESS IN NURSING**: Making the Most of Mentoring *(Vance)*

Fast Facts for the **CATH LAB NURSE** *(McCulloch)*

Fast Facts for the **CLASSROOM NURSING INSTRUCTOR**: Classroom Teaching *(Yoder-Wise, Kowalski)*

Fast Facts for the **CLINICAL NURSE LEADER** *(Wilcox, Deerhake)*

Fast Facts for the **CLINICAL NURSE MANAGER**: Managing a Changing Workplace, Second Edition *(Fry)*

Fast Facts for the **CLINICAL NURSING INSTRUCTOR**: Clinical Teaching, Third Edition *(Kan, Stabler-Haas)*

Fast Facts on **COMBATING NURSE BULLYING, INCIVILITY, AND WORKPLACE VIOLENCE**: What Nurses Need to Know *(Ciocco)*

Fast Facts About **COMPETENCY-BASED EDUCATION IN NURSING**: How to Teach Competency Mastery *(Wittmann-Price, Gittings)*

Fast Facts for the **CRITICAL CARE NURSE**, Second Edition *(Hewett)*

Fast Facts About **CURRICULUM DEVELOPMENT IN NURSING**: How to Develop and Evaluate Educational Programs, Second Edition *(McCoy, Anema)*

Fast Facts for **DEMENTIA CARE**: What Nurses Need to Know, Second Edition *(Miller)*

Fast Facts for **DEVELOPING A NURSING ACADEMIC PORTFOLIO**: What You Really Need to Know *(Wittmann-Price)*

Fast Facts for **DNP ROLE DEVELOPMENT**: A Career Navigation Guide *(Menonna-Quinn, Tortorella Genova)*

Fast Facts About **EKGs FOR NURSES**: The Rules of Identifying EKGs *(Landrum)*

Fast Facts for the **ER NURSE**: Guide to a Successful Emergency Department Orientation, Fourth Edition *(Buettner)*

Fast Facts for **EVIDENCE-BASED PRACTICE IN NURSING**: Third Edition *(Godshall)*

Fast Facts for the **FAITH COMMUNITY NURSE**: Implementing FCN/Parish Nursing *(Hickman)*

Fast Facts About **FORENSIC NURSING**: What You Need to Know *(Scannell)*

Fast Facts for the **GERONTOLOGY NURSE**: A Nursing Care Guide *(Eliopoulos)*

Fast Facts About **GI AND LIVER DISEASES FOR NURSES**: What APRNs Need to Know *(Chaney)*

Fast Facts About the **GYNECOLOGICAL EXAM**: A Professional Guide for NPs, PAs, and Midwives, Second Edition *(Secor, Fantasia)*

Fast Facts in **HEALTH INFORMATICS FOR NURSES** *(Hardy)*

Fast Facts for **HEALTH PROMOTION IN NURSING**: Promoting Wellness *(Miller)*

Fast Facts for Nurses About **HOME INFUSION THERAPY**: The Expert's Best Practice Guide *(Gorski)*

Fast Facts for the **HOSPICE NURSE**: A Concise Guide to End-of-Life Care, Second Edition *(Wright)*

Fast Facts for the **L&D NURSE**: Labor & Delivery Orientation, Second Edition *(Groll)*

Fast Facts About **LGBTQ CARE FOR NURSES** *(Traister)*

Fast Facts for the **LONG-TERM CARE NURSE**: What Nursing Home and Assisted Living Nurses Need to Know *(Eliopoulos)*

Fast Facts to **LOVING YOUR RESEARCH PROJECT**: A Stress-Free Guide for Novice Researchers in Nursing and Healthcare *(Marshall)*

Fast Facts for **MAKING THE MOST OF YOUR CAREER IN NURSING** *(Redulla)*

Fast Facts for **MANAGING PATIENTS WITH A PSYCHIATRIC DISORDER**: What RNs, NPs, and New Psych Nurses Need to Know *(Marshall)*

Fast Facts About **MEDICAL CANNABIS AND OPIOIDS**: Minimizing Opioid Use Through Cannabis *(Smith, Smith)*

Fast Facts for the **MEDICAL OFFICE NURSE**: What You Really Need to Know *(Richmeier)*

Fast Facts for the **MEDICAL–SURGICAL NURSE**: Clinical Orientation (*Ciocco*)

Fast Facts for the **NEONATAL NURSE**: Care Essentials for Normal and High-Risk Neonates, Second Edition (*Davidson*)

Fast Facts About **NEUROCRITICAL CARE**: A Quick Reference for the Advanced Practice Provider (*McLaughlin*)

Fast Facts for the **NEW NURSE PRACTITIONER**: What You Really Need to Know, Second Edition (*Aktan*)

Fast Facts for **NURSE PRACTITIONERS:** Practice Essentials for Clinical Subspecialties (*Aktan*)

Fast Facts for the **NURSE PRECEPTOR**: Keys to Providing a Successful Preceptorship, Second Edition (*Ciocco*)

Fast Facts for the **NURSE PSYCHOTHERAPIST**: The Process of Becoming (*Jones, Tusaie*)

Fast Facts About **NURSING AND THE LAW**: Law for Nurses (*Grant, Ballard*)

Fast Facts About the **NURSING PROFESSION**: Historical Perspectives (*Hunt*)

Fast Facts for the **OPERATING ROOM NURSE**: An Orientation and Care Guide, Third Edition (*Criscitelli*)

Fast Facts for the **PEDIATRIC NURSE**: An Orientation Guide (*Rupert, Young*)

Fast Facts Handbook for **PEDIATRIC PRIMARY CARE:** A Guide for Nurse Practitioners and Physician Assistants (*Ruggiero, Ruggiero*)

Fast Facts About **PRESSURE ULCER CARE FOR NURSES**: How to Prevent, Detect, and Resolve Them (*Dziedzic*)

Fast Facts About **PTSD**: A Guide for Nurses and Other Health Care Professionals (*Adams*)

Fast Facts for the **RADIOLOGY NURSE**: An Orientation and Nursing Care Guide, Second Edition (*Grossman*)

Fast Facts About **RELIGION FOR NURSES**: Implications for Patient Care (*Taylor*)

Fast Facts for the **SCHOOL NURSE**: What You Need to Know, Third Edition (*Loschiavo*)

Fast Facts About **SEXUALLY TRANSMITTED INFECTIONS**: A Nurse's Guide to Expert Patient Care (*Scannell*)

Fast Facts for **STROKE CARE NURSING**: An Expert Care Guide, Second Edition (*Morrison*)

Fast Facts for the **STUDENT NURSE**: Nursing Student Success (*Stabler-Haas*)

Fast Facts About **SUBSTANCE USE DISORDERS**: What Every Nurse, APRN, and PA Needs to Know (*Marshall, Spencer*)

Fast Facts for the **TRAVEL NURSE**: Travel Nursing (*Landrum*)

Fast Facts for the **TRIAGE NURSE**: An Orientation and Care Guide, Second Edition (*Visser, Montejano*)

Fast Facts for **WOUND CARE NURSING**: Practical Wound Management, Second Edition (*Myers*)

Fast Facts for **WRITING THE DNP PROJECT**: Effective Structure, Content, and Presentation (*Christenbery*)

Forthcoming FAST FACTS Books

Fast Facts for the **ADULT-GERONTOLOGY ACUTE CARE NURSE PRACTITIONER** (*Carpenter*)

Fast Facts About **DIVERSITY, EQUITY, AND INCLUSION** (*Davis*)

Fast Facts for the **L&D NURSE**: Labor & Delivery Orientation, Third Edition (*Groll*)

Fast Facts for **PATIENT SAFETY IN NURSING** (*Hunt*)

Visit www.springerpub.com to order.

FAST FACTS About
LGBTQ+ CARE FOR NURSES

Tyler Traister, DNP, RN-BC, NE-BC, CNE, OCN, CHPN, CTN-A, NPD-BC, is an assistant professor of nursing at the University of Pittsburgh and a clinical staff nurse for the UPMC Health Systems in Pittsburgh, Pennsylvania. His scholarly emphasis and practice focus on improving the health and well-being of LGBTQ people, and he is recognized as a clinical expert in LGBTQ health. He completed his doctoral studies at Carlow University, and his doctoral work on LGBTQ cultural competence has been both published and presented at numerous regional and national conferences. He aims to disrupt the gender binary and heteronormativity in healthcare and nursing. He has received several accolades for his diversity and inclusion efforts.

Dr. Traister's clinical background includes medical–surgical, oncology, and nursing leadership, ranging from staff nurse to unit director; clinical practice; and academia. He holds six national nursing certifications in the following specialties: medical–surgical nursing, nurse executive, oncology certified nurse, hospice and palliative care, nurse educator, advanced transcultural nursing, and nursing professional development.

FAST FACTS About
LGBTQ+ CARE FOR NURSES

Tyler Traister, DNP, RN-BC, NE-BC, CNE, OCN, CHPN, CTN-A, NPD-BC

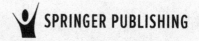

SPRINGER PUBLISHING

Springer Publishing Company, LLC
11 West 42nd Street, New York, NY 10036
www.springerpub.com
connect.springerpub.com/

Acquisitions Editor: Rachel X. Landes
Compositor: Amnet Systems

ISBN: 978-0-8261-6151-2
ebook ISBN: 978-0-8261-6156-7
DOI: 10.1891/9780826161567

Printed by BnT

The author and the publisher of this Work have made every effort to use sources believed to be reliable to provide information that is accurate and compatible with the standards generally accepted at the time of publication. Because medical science is continually advancing, our knowledge base continues to expand. Therefore, as new information becomes available, changes in procedures become necessary. We recommend that the reader always consult current research and specific institutional policies before performing any clinical procedure or delivering any medication. The author and publisher shall not be liable for any special, consequential, or exemplary damages resulting, in whole or in part, from the readers' use of, or reliance on, the information contained in this book. The publisher has no responsibility for the persistence or accuracy of URLs for external or third-party internet websites referred to in this publication and does not guarantee that any content on such websites is, or will remain, accurate or appropriate.

Library of Congress Cataloging-in-Publication Data

Names: Traister, Tyler, author.
Title: Fast facts about LGBTQ+ care for nurses / Tyler Traister.
Other titles: Fast facts (Springer Publishing Company)
Description: New York, NY : Springer Publishing Company, LLC, [2022] |
    Series: Fast facts | Includes bibliographical references and index.
Identifiers: LCCN 2021021486 (print) | LCCN 2021021487 (ebook) | ISBN
    9780826161512 (paperback) | ISBN 9780826161567 (ebook)
Subjects: MESH: Nursing Care—methods | Culturally Competent Care—methods
    | Sexual and Gender Minorities | Education, Nursing | Social Stigma
Classification: LCC RT83.3 (print) | LCC RT83.3 (ebook) | NLM WY 150 |
    DDC 610.73086/6—dc23
LC record available at https://lccn.loc.gov/2021021486
LC ebook record available at https://lccn.loc.gov/2021021487

Publisher's Note: New and used products purchased from third-party sellers are not guaranteed for quality, authenticity, or access to any included digital components.

Printed in the United States of America.

Contents

Preface

I wrote this book to provide nurses from all practice settings and experience levels the knowledge and understanding of how to care for the LGBTQ population. The first of its kind, this book offers the nurse concise and pragmatic information to deliver culturally competent and inclusive care.

LGBTQ and other gender minorities face unique challenges and barriers to accessing healthcare, resulting in poor health outcomes. Studies have consistently shown the greater risk for poor health outcomes due to fear or mistrust of healthcare providers, such as nurses, because of past discrimination and refusal of care and acceptance, which have created systemic health disparities. Nursing textbooks and education predominantly focus on cisgender heteronormative populations—leaving the nurse without the knowledge and information needed to care for this diverse population.

Part I reviews the foundational aspects of caring for LGBTQ people, including definitions and terminology, the basics of culturally competent care, and provides the reader with a deeper understanding of sexuality and gender, while Part II provides the reader with a background and context of LGBTQ health and health disparities.

Part III focuses on the nursing care of this population. Chapter 8 guides the nurse to better understand their self-awareness and biases and lays the foundation to provide culturally competent care. The following chapters discuss critical aspects of caring for patients who identify as LGBTQ and how the nurse can care for them across the life span. Chapter 13 and Chapter 14 provide the nurse with an overview of transgender health and caring for this special population. Each chapter includes case studies to provide the reader with a further understanding and apply them to clinical practice.

Part IV provides and explores resources for nurses and healthcare organizations in caring for LGBTQ people. Chapter 16 highlights how first encounters often set the stage for a positive experience and how we can create a welcoming and inclusive environment. The reader will learn about the impact of policy and legal issues facing the population in Chapter 17. This chapter has practical tips and guides for nurses to expand their care to advocate for creating inclusive environments, curriculums, and organizations.

This book is an all-in-one reference and guides for nurses. The information is applicable for nurses who work at the bedside to advanced practice roles and even in the executive boardroom. I hope that this text offers nurses the information they need to care for LGBTQ people and to open nursing and healthcare beyond hetero-normativity and gender binary. Together we can create a profession that welcomes all people under the rainbow and a healthier, more accepting world for all.

Tyler Traister

Acknowledgments

For those who have been with me since the beginning and for those that joined along the way—look at what we have made.

To the queer people of the world—this book is for you. From Marsha P. Johnson to our queer youth today—you inspire me to create a better world for us to live and love without fear.

Special thanks to my husband, Craig, and our two dogs, Jackson and Dodge; without their endless amounts of love, support, and fluff, this book would not be possible.

Lastly, I would like to acknowledge Rachel Landes, acquisitions editor at Springer Publishing, who approached me after a conference presentation and discussed the amazing opportunity to create this text. Thank you for your support, patience, and guidance through this endeavor.

1

Understanding LGBTQ

1

The ABCs of LGBTQ

Many terms and letters have been used to describe the LGBTQ communities. Outsiders looking in may feel that the letters are overwhelming, academic, or inaccessible to the rest of the population. The intention of these letters is to give identity to a group that was often just called "the gay community." Although the attempt of the acronym was to be inclusive, the lettering can also be limiting. For the purposes of this book, the acronym LGBTQ is used, but it is by no means a definitive descriptor of the population.

In this chapter, you will learn:

1. The definition of LGBTQ terms and definitions
2. How to use these common terms

LGBTQ EXPLAINED

The language that is used to talk about LGBTQ people continues to evolve and expand. "LGBT" became popular in the late 20th century. The addition and use of the "Q" gained traction as the 20th century turned into the 21st. Many variations of the acronym exist with some gaining popularity in various different settings. It may seem that while new terms are appearing, forgotten or unused terms are becoming mainstream and words once viewed as derogatory are being reclaimed and commonplace.

For nurses, it is important to understand the basics of the language that LGBTQ people use to identify themselves. An example of this evolution is the use of the word "queer." Once a pejorative, many people have reclaimed this word to describe their sexual or gender identity. Understand that although one patient may describe themselves as queer, this term could potentially be divisive to some patients because of its history. LGBTQ people today have a large vocabulary with which they can articulate their gender identity and their sexual orientations. These words can make some nurses and healthcare providers feel uncomfortable.

Fast Facts

By asking, learning, and understanding terminology, abbreviations, and acronyms association with LGBTQ people can help nurses to confront their biases or assumptions and promote culturally competent care.

In nursing and healthcare, it might be common to see the LGBTQ community called *sexual and gender minorities*. Researchers may use sexual orientation and gender identity (SOGI) when referring to data about LGBTQ people. In public health, men who have sex with men (MSM) and women who have sex with women (WSW) may also be used to understand a person's sexual habits without referring to their sexual orientation. Understanding these acronyms and terms can help nurses to understand their patients, become an ally to LGBTQ people, and allow us to facilitate conversations with our patients (see Box 1.1). Most importantly, it is the first step in listening to who patients are as people.

LGBTQ TERMS AND DEFINITIONS

Affirmed gender (*noun*): The gender by which one wishes to be known. This term is often used to replace terms like "new gender" or "chosen gender," which imply that a person's gender was chosen rather than simply innate.

   Agender (*adj.*): Describes a person who does not identify with any gender identity.

   Ally (*noun*): A person who does not identify as LGBTQ but stands with and advocates for LGBTQ people.

   Androgynous (*adj.*), **Androgyne** (*noun*): Used to describe someone who identifies or presents as neither distinguishably masculine nor feminine.

BOX 1.1 LGBTQ DEFINED

- **L (Lesbian):** A *lesbian* is a woman who feels a sexual and romantic attraction to other women.
- **G (Gay):** *Gay* is usually a term used to refer to men who feel sexual and romantic attraction to other men. Lesbians can also be referred to as gay.
- **B (Bisexual):** *Bisexual* indicates having a romantic and sexual attraction to both men and women.
- **T (Transgender):** *Transgender* is a term that indicates that a person's gender identity or expression is different from the sex they were assigned at birth.
- **Q (Queer or Questioning):** This initial usually represents queer or questioning. *Queer* is considered an umbrella term for anyone who is non-cisgender or heterosexual. Queer may be used by people who feel that another term such as *gay*, *lesbian*, or *bisexual* is too limiting or not representative of their identity. Questioning refers to people who may be unsure of their sexual orientation or gender identity.

Other variations:
- **LGBTQIA:** This acronym includes initials for queer, intersex, and asexual.
- **LGBTIQA+:** This variation stands for lesbian, gay, bisexual, transgender, intersex, queer/questioning, asexual, and others that can include pansexual and nonbinary.

Sources: GLAAD & HRC.

Aromantic (*adj.*): A romantic orientation generally characterized by not feeling romantic attraction or a desire for romance.

Asexual (*adj.*): Used to describe people who do not experience sexual attraction or do not have a desire for sex. Many experience romantic or emotional attractions across the entire spectrum of sexual orientations. Asexuality differs from celibacy, which refers to abstaining from sex. Also *ace* or *ace community*.

Assigned sex (*noun*): The sex that is assigned to an infant at birth based on the child's visible sex organs, including genitalia and other physical characteristics. Often corresponds with a child's *assigned gender* and *assumed gender*.

Binary system (*noun*): Something that contains two opposing parts; binary systems are often assumed despite the existence of a spectrum of possibilities. Gender (man/woman) and sex (male/female) are examples of binary systems often perpetuated by our culture.

Biological sex (*noun*): A medical classification that refers to anatomical, physiological, genetic, or physical attributes that determine if a person is assigned male, female, or intersex identity at birth. Biological sex is often confused or interchanged with the term "gender," which encompasses personal identity and social factors, and is not necessarily determined by biological sex. See *gender.*

Cisgender (*adj.*): Describes a person whose gender identity (*defined later in this section*) aligns with the sex assigned to them at birth.

Cissexism (*noun*): A system of discrimination and exclusion that oppresses people whose gender and/or gender expression falls outside of normative social constructs. This system is founded on the belief that there are, and should be, only two genders—usually tied to assigned sex.

Coming out (*verb*): A lifelong process of self-acceptance and revealing one's queer identity to others. This may involve something as private as telling a single confidant or something as public as posting to social media.

Demisexual (*adj.*): Used to describe someone who feels sexual attraction only to people with whom they have an emotional bond—often considered to be on the asexual spectrum.

Gender (*noun*): A set of social, physical, psychological, and emotional traits, often influenced by societal expectations, that classify an individual as feminine, masculine, androgynous, or other. Words and qualities ascribed to these traits vary across cultures.

Gender dysphoria (*noun*): Clinically significant distress caused when a person's assigned birth gender is not the same as the one with which they identify.

Gender expression (*noun*): External appearance of one's gender identity, usually expressed through behavior, clothing, haircut, or voice, which may or may not conform to socially defined behaviors and characteristics typically associated with being masculine or feminine.

Gender-fluid (*adj.*): A person who does not identify with a single fixed gender and whose identification and presentation may shift, whether within or outside of the male/female binary.

Gender identity (*noun*): One's innermost feeling of maleness, femaleness, a blend of both, or neither. One's gender identity can be the same or different from their sex assigned at birth.

Gender-neutral (*adj.*): Not gendered, usually operating outside the male/female binary. Can refer to language (e.g., pronouns), spaces (e.g., bathrooms), or identities.

Gender nonconforming (*adj.*): A broad term referring to people who do not behave in a way that conforms to the traditional expectations of their gender or whose gender expression does not fit neatly into a category.

Genderqueer (*adj.*): Describes a person who rejects static categories of gender (i.e., the gender binary of male/female) and whose gender expression or identity falls outside of the dominant social norms of their assigned sex. They may identify as having aspects of both male and female identities or neither.

Gender roles (*noun*): The social behaviors and expression that a culture expects from people based on their assigned sex (e.g., girls wear pink; boys do not cry; women care for home and child; men are more violent), despite a spectrum of various other possibilities.

Heteronormativity (*noun*): Coined by social critic Michael Warner, the term refers to a societal assumption of certain norms:

1. There are two distinct sexes.
2. Male and female functions and characteristics are distinctly different.
3. Traits such as attraction and sexual behavior correspond to anatomy.

Those who do not fit these norms—be it through same-sex attraction, a nonbinary gender identity, or nontraditional gender expression—are therefore seen as *abnormal* and often marginalized or pressured to conform to norms as a result.

Heterosexism (*noun*): The assumption that sexuality between people of different sexes is normal, standard, superior, or universal while other sexual orientations are substandard, inferior, abnormal, marginal, or invalid.

Heterosexual (*adj.*): Used to describe people whose enduring physical, romantic, and/or emotional attraction is to people of the opposite sex. Also *straight*.

Heterosexual/cisgender privilege (*noun*): Refers to societal advantages that heterosexual people and cisgender people have solely because of their dominant identities. This can include things as simple as safely holding hands with a romantic partner in public or having safe access to public bathrooms. This can also include systemic privileges such as the right to legally donate blood, to adopt children without facing possible rejection because of your sexual orientation, or to play organized sports with others of the same gender identity.

Homophobia (*noun*): A fear or hostility toward lesbian, gay, and/or bisexual people, often expressed as discrimination, harassment, and violence.

Intersex (*adj.*): An umbrella term describing people born with reproductive or sexual anatomy and/or a chromosome pattern that cannot be classified as typically male or female.

Latinx (*adj.*): A gender-expansive term for people of Latin American descent used to be more inclusive of all genders than the binary terms Latino or Latina.

Misgender (*verb*): To refer to someone in a way that does not correctly reflect the gender with which they identify, such as refusing to use a person's pronouns or name.

Nonbinary (*adj.*): An umbrella term that refers to individuals who identify as neither man or woman, or as a combination of man or woman. Instead, nonbinary people exhibit a boundless range of identities that can exist beyond a spectrum between male and female.

Outing (*verb*): The inappropriate act of publicly declaring (sometimes based on rumor and/or speculation) or revealing another person's sexual orientation or gender identity without that person's consent.

Pansexual (*adj.*): Used to describe people who have the potential for emotional, romantic, or sexual attraction to people of any gender identity, though not necessarily simultaneously, in the same way, or to the same degree. The term *panromantic* may refer to a person who feels these emotional and romantic attractions but identifies as asexual.

Preferred pronouns (*adj.*): The pronoun or set of pronouns that an individual personally uses and would like others to use when talking to or about that individual. Can include variations of *he/him/his*, *she/her/hers*, and *they/their/theirs*, among others. This term is being used less and less in LGBTQ circles, as it suggests one's gender identity is a "preference" rather than innate. *Recommended replacement: "Your pronouns, my pronouns, their pronouns, and so forth."*

Queer (*adj.*): Once a pejorative term, a term reclaimed and used by some within academic circles and the LGBTQ community to describe sexual orientations and gender identities that are not exclusively heterosexual or cisgender.

Questioning (*adj.*): A term used to describe people who are in the process of exploring their sexual orientation or gender identity.

Same-gender loving (*adj.*): This term was and is used by some members of the Black community who feel that terms like *gay, lesbian,* and *bisexual* (and sometimes the communities therein) are Eurocentric and fail to affirm Black culture, history, and identity.

Sexual orientation (*noun*): An inherent or immutable emotional, romantic, or sexual attraction to other people; oftentimes used to signify the gender identity (or identities) to which a person is most attracted.

Third gender (*noun*): A gender identity that is neither male nor female, existing outside the idea that gender represents a linear spectrum between the two. Sometimes a catchall term or category in societies, states, or countries that legally recognize genders other than male and female.

Transgender (*adj.*): An umbrella term for people whose gender identity differs from the sex they were assigned at birth. Not all trans people undergo transition. Being transgender does not imply any specific sexual orientation. Therefore, transgender people may identify as straight, gay, lesbian, bisexual, or something else. Also, *trans*.

Transitioning (*verb*): A process during which some people strive to more closely align their gender identity with their gender expression. This includes *socially transitioning*, during which a person may change their pronouns, the name they ask to be called, or the way they dress to be socially recognized as another gender. This includes *legal transitioning*, which may involve an official name change and modified IDs and birth certificates. And this includes *physically transitioning*, during which a person may undergo medical interventions to more closely align their body to their gender identity. Transgender and nonbinary people transition in various ways to various degrees; self-identification alone is enough to validate gender identity.

Transphobia (*noun*): The fear and hatred of, or discomfort with, transgender people. This may manifest into transphobic actions, such as violence, harassment, misrepresentation, or exclusion.

Transsexual (*adj.*): A less frequently used term (considered by some to be outdated or offensive), which refers to people who use medical interventions such as hormone therapy, gender-affirming surgery (GAS), or sex reassignment surgery (SRS) as part of the process of expressing their gender. Some people who identify as transsexual do not identify as transgender and vice versa. *Only use this term if someone who specifically identifies as such asks you to.*

Two spirit (*adj.*): An umbrella term in Native culture to describe people who have both a male and female spirit within them. This encompasses many tribe-specific names, roles, and traditions, such as the *winkte* of the Lakota and *nadleeh* of the Navajo people. This term often describes Native people who performed roles and gender expression associated with both men and women. *This term should be used only in the context of Native culture.*

Words are important to LGBTQ people as they can provide a person with a sense of identity and a way to describe themselves. However, they can also be limiting and not capture the full identity of the diverse population that is the LGBTQ population. Nurses should have a basic understanding of the various terms and vocabulary surrounding LGBTQ people so they are able to better understand and listen to their patients.

Further Reading

GLAAD Media Reference Guide—Lesbian/gay/bisexual glossary of terms. (2016, October 26). Retrieved January 15, 2021, from https://www.glaad.org/reference/lgbtq

Gold, M. (2018, June 21). *The ABCs of L.G.B.T.Q.I.A.+*. Retrieved January 15, 2021, from https://www.nytimes.com/2018/06/21/style/lgbtq-gender-language.html

Human Rights Campaign. (n.d.). *Glossary of terms*. Retrieved January 15, 2021, from https://www.hrc.org/resources/glossary-of-terms

LGBTQ+ glossary. (n.d.). Retrieved January 15, 2021, from https://health.ucdavis.edu/diversity-inclusion/LGBTQI/LGBTQ-Plus.html

Mayer, K. H., Potter, J., Goldhammer, H., & Makadon, H. J. (2015). *The Fenway guide to lesbian, gay, bisexual, and transgender health*. American College of Physicians.

2

Brief History of LGBTQ

LGBTQ people are found throughout history. The idea of same-sex couples and gender-variant people is not a contemporary issue that arose in recent years. They are interwoven in cultures across the globe and represented in stories and artwork. Many famous figures from ancient to modern history are rumored as or identify as LGBTQ. This chapter provides the nurse with the historical background of LGBTQ people. Having this insight will allow the nurse to appreciate LGBTQ people and their presence better and understand how LGBTQ people live in our country today.

In this chapter, you will learn:

1. Historical highlights of the LGBTQ community
2. How LGBTQ history plays a role in their current health and well-being
3. Why LGBTQ history is vital to the nurse

LGBTQ PEOPLE IN GLOBAL HISTORY

Almost all ancient civilizations have recorded instances of same sex and sexuality. Furthermore, the concept and history of a third gender, including those who could be considered intersex or gender fluid, have been well represented worldwide.

Americas

- Before the colonization of North America by Europeans, the Americas' Indigenous people had respected roles for people now known as LGBTQ.
  - Many of these roles are revered and are spiritual or social.
- Each tribal nation or culture had their unique name for these individuals.
- The term *two spirited* became popular in the 1990s.
  - Two-spirit people combined activities of both men and women with traits unique to their status as two-spirit people. In most tribes, they were considered neither men nor women and considered a unique and alternative gender (Indian Health Services, 2020).

Asia, India, and Africa

- Many famous Chinese and Japanese works of literature mentioned homosexuality or gender identity.
- Many Hindu and Vedic textual works contain various saints and demigods who possessed multiple sexes and gender combinations (Halsall, 2020).
- The ancient text of Kama Sutra describes homosexual practices and ideas of sex and gender in several places throughout (HRC, 2020).
- Egyptian history has some of the earliest mentions and depictions of same-sex relationships (Burton, 2020).

Ancient Greek and Roman

- Perhaps some of the most representative of LGBTQ people arise from Greek and Roman literature and art.
  - Having both male and female physical relationships was a cultural norm in Ancient Greece.
- Alexander the Great
  - Maybe the world's most notable bisexual. Many historical texts have portrayed Alexander as a heterosexual; however, this is believed to have erased his bisexuality to fit subsequent cultures' norms (Kitchen, 2020).

European History

- Sexual and gender diversity was present during the medieval to the modern period in Europe.
  - Expanding religious dogmas and nationalism introduced new laws and punishments against same-sex sexual acts.

- Migration and conquest played a role in the variance of acceptance throughout eras.
- The Catholic Inquisition saw large numbers of homosexual people murdered (Monro, 2015).
- Rumored gay people of this time include Leonardo daVinci and Michelangelo and many people of nobility (Ogles, 2016).
- France became the first European country to decriminalize sodomy in 1791.

TERMINOLOGY THROUGH THE TIMES

19th Century

- Developments in psychology, led primarily by Richard von Krafft-Ebing and Havelock Ellis, allowed homosexuality to be addressed outside of religion.
  - During this time, men and women attracted to the same sex and those whose gender identity did not match their birth sex were considered "sexual deviants."
  - The transition from the use of "sodomy" and "sodomites" to "homosexuality."
    - Instead of a negative "act," now a human trait or part of our identity.
  - Homosexuality during this time was considered an inherent disposition of "degeneracy."
    - Many theories that homosexuality derived from moral, physical, or intellectual abnormalities.
      - Symptoms of disease, malnourishment, alcohol, and other failures of society.

20th Century

- The term *homosexual* gained popularity in the 20th century.
  - Broad term and did not make distinctions.
  - Advocates attempted to change the term to *homophile* to remove the emphasis on "sexual."
- *Gay* gained traction as a synonym for *homosexuals* in the early 20th century.
  - During this time, the term encompassed men, lesbians, bisexuals, and people who would later be called transgender.
  - The 1970s brought this term from the underground into the mainstream.
- A rise in feminism and activism during the 1970s later prompted women the want and desire to distinguish themselves

from their male counterparts; thus, the term *lesbian* gained popularity.

- *Gay and lesbian* became an umbrella term for the LGBTQ population in 1980 and included transgender people.
- In the late 1990s, the acronym LGBT came into use and was meant to be inclusive.
- The 21st century brought increasing visibility to transgender people, sexual orientation, and gender diversity. In response to that, many groups expanded the acronym to LGBTQ, and many variations exist today.

Fast Facts

Many nursing organizations have created position statements, panels, and educational resources about LGBTQ health and nurses.

A TIMELINE OF LGBTQ HISTORY IN AMERICA

The movement for LGBTQ rights in America dates back to the 1920s when the first documented gay rights organization was founded: the Society for Human Rights.

1952

- The American Psychiatric Association lists homosexuality in their diagnostic manual as a sociopathic personality disturbance.
- Christine Jorgensen is the first American who comes forward publicly about being transgender and speaks openly about her gender confirmation surgery and hormone replacement therapy experiences. For many, she is the first visible transgender person in the media.

1953

- President Eisenhower signs an executive order that bans homosexuals from working for the federal government—citing them as a national security risk.

1956

- The Daughters of Bilitis (DOB) is formed and is considered the first-known lesbian rights organization.

1961

- Illinois is the first state to decriminalize homosexuality by decriminalizing sodomy laws.

1969

- On June 28, 1969, police raid the Stonewall Inn in New York City that resulted in protests and demonstrations.
  - The Stonewall Riots are believed to be the foundation of today's LGBTQ movement.
  - On June 28, 1970, community members in New York City marched to recognize the Stonewall Riots' first anniversary and consider the world's first pride parade.

1973

- The American Psychiatric Association votes to remove homosexuality from its list of mental disorders.

1978

- Harvey Milk is elected as a city supervisor in San Francisco in 1978, becoming the first openly gay man to be elected to public office in California.
- Milk is later assassinated that year. His death leads to the creation of the first rainbow flag.

1979

- On October 14, 1979, the first National March on Washington for Lesbian and Gay Rights takes place.

1982

- Wisconsin becomes the first state to outlaw discrimination on sexual orientation.
- Nearly 800 people are infected with gay-related immunodeficiency disorder (GRID). The name is changed to AIDS by the year's end.

1993

- President Clinton signs a directive prohibiting openly gay and lesbian Americans from serving in the U.S. military through the "Don't Ask, Don't Tell" policy.

1996

- The Defense of Marriage Act is signed into law.
  - This act bans federal same-sex marriage and defines marriage as a legal union between a man and a woman.

1997

- Ellen DeGeneres comes out as a lesbian.

1998

- Matthew Shepard dies on October 12, 1998, after being beaten, tortured, and left to die. Shepard's sexuality was part of the motive for murder by two men.
- Vermont becomes the first state in the country to recognize civil unions between gay and lesbian couples legally.

2003

- The U.S. Supreme Court, with their opinion in *Lawrence v. Texas*, decriminalizes "homosexual conduct."
- The Massachusetts Supreme Court rules that barring gays and lesbians from marrying violated the state constitution.

2004

- On May 17, 2004, the first legal same-sex marriage in the United States occurs in Massachusetts.

2008

- California becomes the second state to legally allow same-sex marriage after a California Supreme Court ruling that states same-sex couples have a constitutional right to marry. This repealed Prop 8, which was a voter-approved proposition.

2009

- President Barack Obama signs the Matthew Shepard and James Byrd Jr. Hate Crimes Prevention Act into Law.

2011

- President Obama repeals Don't Ask, Don't Tell, allowing LGBTQ people to serve openly in the military.

2012

- President Obama is the first sitting U.S. president to support the freedom for LGBTQ people to marry.
- The Democratic Party is the first major political party in the United States to support same-sex marriage publicly.
- Tammy Baldwin is the first open lesbian to be elected in the U.S. Senate.

2013 to 2020

- Over several years, the Supreme Court delivers several landmark rulings that change the landscape of LGBTQ rights in the United States:
  - 2013: *United States v. Windsor*, the U.S. Supreme Court strikes down a section of the Defense of Marriage Act and rules that legally married same-sex couples are entitled to federal benefits.
  - 2015: *Obergefell v. Hodges* is a landmark civil rights case that makes same-sex marriage the law of the land that states cannot ban same-sex marriage.
  - 2020: *Bostock v. Clayton County* is another landmark civil rights case that rules that federal law protects LGBTQ people from discrimination and extends the protections from Title VII of the Civil Rights Act to LGBTQ people (Box 2.1).

Nursing can end the invisibility of LGBTQ in healthcare, but to do that, we have to understand the history of LGBTQ people. With this knowledge, nurses can deliver culturally competent care. In recent years, focus on nursing and healthcare has been placed on LGBTQ people and the health disparities. This is true now more than it was even only a decade ago. Thanks to publications in the last decade like the Joint Commission's "Field Guide" on LGBTQ health, the Institute of Medicine (IOM) report on "Health of Lesbian, Gay, Bisexual, and Transgender People," and the addition of LGBT people into the goals of Healthy People 2020, a highlight and focus have been placed on the existence of health disparities affecting the LGBTQ people.

- One example of how understanding the history of LGBTQ people in our country for nurses is by caring for our veteran population. Only a decade ago, LGBTQ people could not serve in the military unless they hid their identity, leading to a lack of trust and fear of discrimination in healthcare. Surveys have shown that LGBTQ veterans are less likely to disclose their LGBTQ identity to providers, which may be associated with adverse health outcomes/

BOX 2.1 NURSING AND LGBTQ

- The American Nurses Association (ANA) first took an official stance on LGBTQ discrimination in 1978.
  - Adopted a resolution supporting legislation to bar discrimination based on sexual orientation.
- Nursing organizations responded to the HIV/AIDS epidemic in the 1980s by supporting evidence-based approaches to controlling the epidemic and opposing discrimination against HIV/AIDS people.
  - In the early days of the HIV/AIDs epidemic, this required nurses to confront the antigay bias.
- The ANA opposed policies barring gay and lesbian individuals from serving in the U.S. military in 1992.
- After the military's ban on gay and lesbian service members was modified into a "Don't Ask, Don't Tell" Policy, the ANA supported efforts to repeal that policy, which was later ended in 2016.
- In 2017, executive attempts to create a ban on transgender individuals serving in the military were unsuccessful. The ANA again advocated in support of equality and human rights for LGBTQ people.

Source: American Nurses Association. (2020). *Nursing advocacy for LGBTQ+ populations: Position statement.* https://www.nursingworld.org/~49866e/global assets/practiceandpolicy/ethics/nursing-advocacy-for-lgbtq-populations.pdf

behaviors. Veterans of this era are also at risk of developing internalized homophobia, self-esteem issues, and identity crises. For nurses, knowing LGBTQ history when caring for our veterans can help us to provide culturally competent care better. Through this knowledge, we can empathize with our patients and honestly care for them as a whole person.

The nurse–patient relationship is at the core of healthcare. Nurses must advocate for and continue to improve the healthcare of LGBTQ people. Understanding their history is the first step. With this knowledge and understanding of LGBTQ history, nurses can practice compassion and respect for all individuals' human rights.

Fast Facts

LGBTQ people are not modern-day development. They are people who have been present throughout human history; often, they are making history.

Further Reading

Aldrich, R. (2020, May 29). *Historical views of homosexuality: European Colonialism.* Oxford Research Encyclopedia of Politics. https://oxfordre .com/politics/view/10.1093/acrefore/9780190228637.001.0001/acrefore -9780190228637-e-1246

American Nurses Association. (2020). *Nursing advocacy for LGBTQ+ populations: Position statement.* https://www.nursingworld.org/~49866e/ globalassets/practiceandpolicy/ethics/nursing-advocacy-for-lgbtq-popu lations.pdf

Bennington-Castro, J. (2019, June 12). *The Supreme Court rulings that have shaped gay rights in America.* https://www.history.com/news/supreme -court-cases-gay-lgbt-rights

Burton, N. (2020). *Meet the gays of ancient Egypt.* https://www.audacy .com/podcasts/pride-23240/meet-the-gays-of-ancient-egypt-w-dr-neel -burton-294250878

Human Rights Campaign. (2020). *Stances of faiths on LGBTQ issues: Hinduism.* https://www.hrc.org/resources/stances-of-faiths-on-lgbt-issues-hinduism

Indian Health Services. (2020). *Health resources.* https://www.ihs.gov/lgbt/ health/twospirit/

Institute of Medicine (US) Committee on Lesbian, Gay, Bisexual, and Transgender Health Issues and Research Gaps and Opportunities. (2011). Context for LGBT Health Status in the United States. In *The health of lesbian, gay, bisexual, and transgender people: Building a foundation for better understanding.* National Academies Press. https://www.ncbi.nlm .nih.gov/books/NBK64801/

The Joint Commission. (2011). *Advancing effective communication, cultural competence, and patient- and family-centered care for the lesbian, gay, bisexual, and transgender (LGBT) community: A field guide.* https://www .jointcommission.org/-/media/tjc/documents/resources/patient-safety -topics/health-equity/lgbtfieldguide_web_linked_verpdf.pdf?db=web& hash=FD725DC02CFE6E4F21A35EBD839BBE97

Kitchen, M. (2020). Interpreting Alexander III of Macedon's "Sexuality" in the Ancient Greco-Macedonian World. *Western Illinois Historical Review.* http://www.wiu.edu/cas/history/wihr/pdfs/WIHR%20spring%202020% 20Kitchen%20final%20version.pdf

LGBTQ history. (n.d.). Retrieved January 15, 2021, from https://www.glsen .org/lgbtq-history

LGBTQ rights milestones fast facts. (2020, December 2). https://www.cnn
.com/2015/06/19/us/lgbt-rights-milestones-fast-facts/index.html

Martos, A. J., Wilson, P. A., & Meyer, I. H. (2017). Lesbian, gay, bisexual, and
transgender (LGBT) health services in the United States: Origins, evolution, and contemporary landscape. *PLoS One, 12*(7), e0180544. https://
doi.org/10.1371/journal.pone.0180544

Monro, S. (2015). LGBT/queer sexuality, history of, Europe. In *The
International Encyclopedia of Human Sexuality.* https://doi.org/10.1002/
9781118896877.wbiehs268

Ogles, J. (2016, October 21). *15 gay romances of the Renaissance era.* Advocate.
https://www.advocate.com/arts-entertainment/2016/10/21/15-gay
-romances-renaissance-era?pg=2&TB_iframe=true&width=850&caption
=Advocate.com&keepThis=true&height=650

Ruben, M. A., Livingston, N. A., Berke, D. S., Matza, A. R., & Shipherd, J. C.
(2019). Lesbian, gay, bisexual, and transgender veterans' experiences of
discrimination in health care and their relation to health outcomes: A
pilot study examining the moderating role of provider communication.
Health Equity, 3(1), 480–488. https://doi.org/10.1089/heq.2019.0069

3

Understanding Sexual Orientation and Gender Identity

This chapter will explore the concepts of sexual orientation and gender identity. Understanding these concepts will help the nurse better understand the lives of LGBTQ. Both are an inherent and immutable aspect of human beings and are an essential part of who we are as people.

In this chapter, you will learn:

1. The basis of sexual orientation and gender identity
2. The importance of collecting sexual orientation and gender identity information in healthcare
3. What it means for LGBTQ people to come out and how the nurse can support them

SEXUAL ORIENTATION

A Definition

Every person has a sexual orientation. *Sexual orientation* refers to an enduring pattern of emotions, romantic, and/or sexual attractions to men, women, or both sexes (American Psychological Association [APA], 2021). A person's sexual orientation can also refer to their

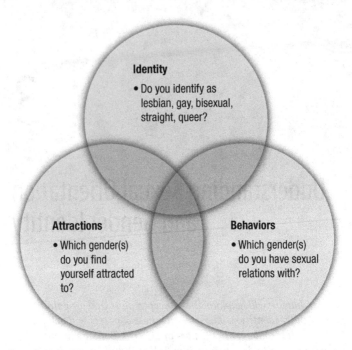

Figure 3.1 Three dimensions of sexual orientation.
Source: Adapted from Fenway Institute.

sense of identity based on those attractions, related behaviors, and membership in a community of others who are similar (see Figure 3.1).

Sexual orientation ranges along a continuum that a person may experience different points throughout their lives. There will be people who are exclusively attracted to the opposite sex and those who are solely attracted to the same sex; however, there are people who exist along that continuum. Sexual orientation should be viewed as fluid in nature and that a person may change over time.

In the context of the lesbian, gay, bisexual, transgender, and queer (LGBTQ acronym), sexual orientation commonly refers to the "LGB." When discussing sexual orientation, it is common to see three categories (see Table 3.1).

As sexual orientation exists on a continuum, some people may use different labels or none at all. Throughout the world, many cultures and nations have terms and descriptions for sexual orientation—with many using various identity labels. For a list of other terms that are used to describe sexual orientation, please refer to Chapter 1.

Table 3.1

LGB Categories	
Orientation	**Definition**
Heterosexual	Having emotional, romantic, or sexual attractions to members of the other sex
Gay/lesbian	Having emotional, romantic, or sexual interests in members of one's sex
Bisexual	Having emotional, romantic, or sexual attractions to both men and women

Fast Facts

Sexual orientation is a separate entity from sex and gender.

Nurses and other healthcare providers assume that sexual orientation is a sole characteristic of a person, such as their age, race, or sex. People express their sexual orientation through various behaviors such as kissing, holding hands, and other intimate acts. Sexual orientation also encompasses nonsexual affections such as shared goals and values, mutual support, and an ongoing commitment to each other. Therefore, sexual orientation should not be seen as a personal characteristic. A person's sexual orientation defines a group of people. That person is likely to find satisfying and fulfilling romantic relationships that are an essential component of personal identity for many people (APA, 2021). Instead of an individual's characteristic, view sexual orientation as a broad concept that is interrelated with a person's relationship with others.

A UNIQUE PROCESS

Stigma and discrimination in our society and culture can make it difficult for many people to come to terms with their sexual orientation. Support patients to come to terms with their sexual orientation on their terms and understand that it a unique process that is individual to each person.

- A person's sexual orientation may start to emerge in middle childhood and into early adolescence.

- Sexual attraction and the associated emotional and romantic responses may arise without any prior sexual experience.
  - People can be celibate and still have a sense or know their sexual orientation.
- Each journey is unique to each person.
  - Every lesbian, gay, and bisexual person has a different experience regarding their sexual orientation.
- Some know their sexual orientation long before pursuing a relationship with other people. In comparison, others may engage in sexual activity (with same sex or opposite) before assigning a label to their sexual orientation.

Researchers have arrived at no consensus on why an individual develops a particular sexual orientation, whether heterosexual, lesbian, gay, or bisexual. Scientists have studied genetic, hormonal development, and social and cultural influences, and there are no conclusive findings that any particular factor or factors determine sexual orientation. Most people experience little or no sense of choice or control about their sexual orientation.

Sexual Orientations Are Not Disorders

Nurses must understand that lesbian, gay, bisexual, and other sexual orientations are not disorders.

- Research has found no association between any sexual orientation and psychopathology.
- Same-sex and opposite-sex behaviors are normal aspects of a human's sexuality.
- Cultures throughout time and across the globe have depictions and documentation of sexual behaviors.

The American Psychiatric Association (APA) removed homosexuality from the *Diagnostic and Statistical Manual of Mental Health (DSM)* in 1973 and has since maintained that homosexuality is not a mental disorder. All mainstream medical and mental health organizations in the United States have concluded that these various orientations represent typical human experience forms. Nurses can help combat the stigma and discrimination faced by LGBTQ people by normalizing lesbian, gay, bisexual, and other sexual orientations.

Fast Facts

Every person has a sexual orientation and gender identity.

GENDER IDENTITY

Sex Versus Gender: What Is the Difference?

Nurses need to understand the critical differences between the terms sex and gender. This understanding is key to nurses delivering culturally congruent care to gender-diverse patients.

Sex is defined as *the traits that distinguish between males and females. Sex refers primarily to physical and biological traits.*

Gender is defined as *the condition of being male, female, or neuter.*

Sex and gender vary in that sex refers to the biological aspects of maleness and femaleness. In contrast, gender implies the psychological, behavioral, social, and cultural aspects of being male or female (i.e., masculinity or femininity; APA, 2021).

Gender as a Spectrum

Note that gender and sex cannot be used interchangeably. The previous definitions show that they are distinct concepts. Aspects of biological sex are similar across different cultures; aspects of gender may differ. Gender is not inherently connected to one's physical anatomy. In Western societies, such as the United States, healthcare organizations and people view gender as a *binary* concept, that a person is either male or female. However, a binary concept of gender fails to recognize or validate the variations of gender that have been and continue to be observed worldwide. Viewing gender as a spectrum and existing along a continuum enables nurses to appreciate a truly authentic model of gender in our patients and people everywhere.

Fast Facts

Sex and gender vary in that sex refers to the biological aspects of maleness and femaleness, whereas gender implies the psychological, behavioral, social, and cultural aspects of being male or female.

Gender is found all around us. Gender expectations and roles are taught to us from birth. Even professions, such as nursing, have been gendered, and men in nursing find themselves challenging the construct of gender in their profession. Many of our gender roles and expectations are ingrained in our culture, in toys, colors, behaviors, and many other aspects of our lives. The concept and various factors of gender profoundly influence our everyday lives, and many people cannot imagine navigating the world in any other way. Individuals who fit into these expectations find they rarely have to question what gender means to them and others. Nurses must understand the role of gender in our society and how some people may exist outside of our society's norms. These people may face challenges, and by understanding the uniqueness and validity of each person's experiences of gender, we can provide them with culturally congruent nursing care.

Dimensions of Gender Identity

Gender identity is further defined by gender as a person's internal sense of gender. Like sexual orientation, gender identity is self-identified and is the result of a combination of inherent and environmental factors (see Figure 3.2). A person may begin to develop feelings about their gender identity as early as age 2 or 3.

Most people will identify as either male or female. Some may feel that they are more masculine or feminine yet still identify as male or female. Others may identify as neither. Terms that these people may use to describe themselves are *genderqueer, gender variant,* or *gender fluid.*

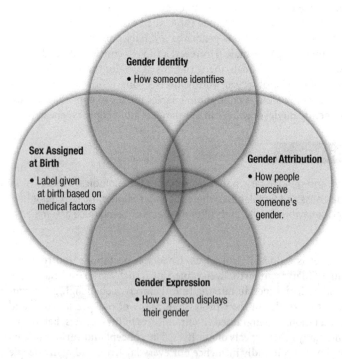

Figure 3.2 Four intersecting domains of gender identity.

- For example, if a person considers himself a male and is most comfortable referring to his gender in masculine terms, then his gender identity is male.
- A person whose assigned sex and gender identity align is called *cisgender*.
- A person whose assigned sex is of the other gender from their gender identity is called *transgender* or *trans*.
- *Assigned sex, sex assigned at birth,* or *biological sex* refers to the label given to people at birth. It is primarily associated with physical attributes such as chromosomes, hormones, and anatomy.

Transgender People

Similar to sexual orientation, there are no singular explanations for why some people are transgender. The wide range of transgender expressions and experiences argue against any one answer. Many experts believe that biological factors such as genetics and prenatal hormone levels, early experiences, and experiences later in adolescence or adulthood may contribute to transgender identities.

Transgender people are often aware of their identity at an earlier age, but they may become aware at any age. Some may remember feelings of "not fitting in" with people of their assigned sex and may have had a desire or specific wishes to be something other than their assigned sex. For some, exploration of their transgender identity may have led to feelings of shame or confusion.

Gender Identity Affirmation

The process in which a transgender person undergoes a social and/or medical transition is commonly referred to transition or gender identity affirmation. Nurses should understand these terms related to transition.

The use of outdated terms such as sexual reassignment surgery can compromise the nurse–patient relationship and invalidate the lived experiences of transgender people. The gender identity affirmation process can be complicated and difficult for some transgender people. This process may include:

- Medical and surgical procedures
- Legal document changes
- Social changes
- Coming out to friends and family
- Reorienting themselves to living in the world in a different gender.

BOX 3.1 TIPS FOR NURSES INTERACTING WITH TRANSGENDER PEOPLE

- Educate yourself about transgender issues through self-learning and discovery.
- Be aware of your biases concerning people with gender-nonconforming appearance or behavior.
- Know that transgender people have membership in various sociocultural identity groups (e.g., race, social class, religion, age, disability). There is not one universal way to look or be transgender.
- Use names and pronouns appropriate to the person's gender presentation and identity.
  - If in doubt, ask.
- Do not make assumptions about transgender people's sexual orientation, desire for hormonal or medical treatment, or other aspects of their identity or transition plans.
- Do not confuse gender nonconformity with being transgender. Not all people who appear androgynous or gender nonconforming identify as transgender or desire gender affirmation treatment.
- Offer support to partners, parents, and children. Validate their concerns and connect them with resources.
- Advocate for transgender rights.

Support transgender people throughout this process and remember that the components of transition are highly individualized. Not all people may need all components, and the order they occur should be flexible to the individual (see Box 3.1).

COMING OUT

The phrase "coming out" is used by LGBT people to describe several aspects of their experiences with their sexual orientation or gender identity. The simplest usage of *coming out* is the experience when an LGBTQ person openly discloses their sexual orientation or gender identity to another person. However, for many LGBTQ people, coming out is a complex process unique to each LGBTQ person. For many, it is the first step in their self-awareness and acceptance of their sexual attractions or gender identity. A person may *come out* with widespread disclosure, or some may choose to tell one or a few people about themselves.

Fast Facts

LGTBQ people must make a conscious choice at every encounter with a new person or new environment about whether, when, whom, and how they may wish to disclose themselves.

Nurses should understand that *coming out* is a gradual and life-long process; there are always new people LGBT need to come out to. Nurses can have a powerful and potentially life-altering effect on our patients by being sensitive to LGBTQ patients' needs and understanding the complexity of coming out.

- Beliefs and norms surrounding gender and sexuality differ among cultures, ethnicities, religions, and the country a person resides in, which make the coming out process unique for each individual.
- Most lesbian, gay, and bisexual people realize their sexual orientation during their teenage years or early 20s.
- Some may discover their sexual orientation without any prior sexual activity, while for others, sexual exploration may clarify their sexual orientation.
- Coming out for transgender people may be tricky as it involves exposing one's inner sense of self, changes in gender, appearance, social role, and some, their physical anatomy. Some transgender people can choose the timing of their coming out, while others may be forced to come out by their gender presentation or during their transition.
- LGTBQ people must make a conscious choice at every encounter with a new person or new environment about whether, when, whom, and how they may wish to disclose themselves.

How Nurses Can Help LGBTQ People With Their Coming Out Process

- Remain open to the nonbinary concept of gender and sexuality that some patients may present with.
- Avoid assumptions based on stereotypes.
- Understand that the coming out process is unique to each individual and consider where they may be in their process and how it may impact clinical care and relationships.
  - This might also affect their sense of self, self-care, and the choices that they may make during clinical encounters.

- ▪ Some people who have difficulty coming out may have maladaptive coping and may engage in high-risk behaviors such as drug and alcohol abuse, sexual promiscuity, and other self-destructive behaviors.
- Develop an awareness of how race, ethnicity, and religion can play a role in a person's coming out process.
- Listen to how patients describe themselves, their partners, and their body. Mirror their language.
- Communicate that being LGBTQ are healthy, normal, and positive expressions of gender and sexuality.
- Always remain positive and affirming when discussing topics of sexuality and gender identity.
- Have resources available for LGBTQ patients, including referrals to LGBTQ affirmative support groups, community organizations, and specialized behavioral health and healthcare providers. Include resources for friends and family members of LGBTQ patients and how they can be supportive.

Further Reading

American Psychological Association. (2021). *Definitions related to sexual orientation and gender diversity in APA documents.*

Dawson, J. (2018). *This book is gay.* Hot Key Books.

Faderman, L. (2016). *The gay revolution the story of the struggle.* Simon & Schuster Paperbacks.

Mayer, K. H., Potter, J., Goldhammer, H., & Makadon, H. J. (2015). *The Fenway guide to lesbian, gay, bisexual, and transgender health.* American College of Physicians.

National LGBTQIA+ Health Education Center. (2020, August 19). *Foundations of LGBTQIA+ health.* https://www.lgbtqiahealtheducation.org/

Parenthood, P. (2021). *Sex and gender identity.* https://www.plannedparenthood.org/learn/gender-identity/sex-gender-identity

PFLAG & Gender Spectrum. (2012). *Understanding gender.* http://www.pflagsf.org/wp-content/uploads/2012/12/Understanding_Gender.pdf

Wharton, A. S. (2012). *The sociology of gender: An introduction to theory and research* (2nd ed.). Wiley-Blackwell.

4

LGBTQ Cultural Competence

Culturally competent care includes the knowledge, attitudes, and skills that can support caring for diverse populations such as LGBTQ people. Cultural competence is a lifelong journey as our world continues to grow and populations become more diverse. This chapter explores the concept of cultural competence, the connection to LGBTQ people, and how the nurse can integrate cultural competence into their care delivery at all levels

In this chapter, you will learn:

1. The importance of cultural competence in caring for LGBTQ people
2. A cultural competence framework to further understand the concept
3. Practical steps in delivering culturally competent care to LGBTQ people
4. How to assess and improve your own level of cultural competency

INTRODUCTION

It could be postulated that in today's society in the United States, cultural competence and understanding are needed now more than ever. With technological advances, we live in an ever-integrating global society that is interconnected in a way that is unlike any other time in our history. Socially, some people may view the urge for cultural competence among healthcare providers to be devalued as a "politically correct manner of behavior or a fad" (Schawewald & Pfeiffer, 2015). However, there are many unfortunate events that happen within our healthcare system that result in injury or even death because of a lack of cultural competence and understanding.

For the LGBTQ population, cultural competence is key to reducing and eliminating health disparities. Negative attitudes and lack of knowledge have been identified as two of the top barriers to LGBTQ culturally competent care (Gendron et al., 2013; Lim et al., 2012; Moone et al., 2016; Strong et al., 2015). A research study revealed that most agencies do not have gender-inclusive forms, nurses were confused on how to assess and communicate with LGBTQ people, and also displayed a lack of knowledge on transgender individuals (Carabez et al., 2015). The negative implications of such findings helped to further affirm their inquiry of institutional erasure and invisibility of transgender people in nursing (Carabez et al., 2015).

Cultural Competence—Defined

- Cultural competence is based on the principles of social justice and human rights (Douglas et al., 2014).
- The International Council of Nurses (ICN) discusses how diversity encompasses acceptance and respect, and for the nurse, this means understanding that each individual is unique and that nursing must recognize individual differences in the people that we serve (ICN, 2013).
  - The ICN defines these differences as spanning the dimensions of race, ethnicity, gender, sexual orientation, social-economic status, age, physical abilities, spiritual or religious beliefs, political beliefs, or other ideologies (ICN, 2013).
- Culturally competent nursing care is a necessary component of care delivery.

Fast Facts

Cultural competence should be viewed as a lifelong process that a person must actively pursue of their own volition.

- Other terms in the literature that were included as a variation of cultural competence are culturally congruent care, cultural safety, and transcultural nursing care.
- By providing culturally competent care, the nurse is able to aid in the reduction of health disparities through patient empowerment, in

the integration of cultural beliefs into healthcare, and by expanding access to healthcare for vulnerable populations (Douglas et al., 2014).

- ■ The U.S. Department of Health and Human Services, Office of Minority Health, states that cultural competence is a matter of national concern.
- ■ Leingener first proposed the theory of transcultural nursing in the 1950s, and subsequently, many models and other theories have arisen as a result of her work (Merryfeather & Bruce, 2014).
- ■ Merryfeather and Bruce operationalize the definition of cultural competence as "beings with an awareness of differences among various cultures, which then develops into personal sensitivity and culminates with the nurse becoming culturally safe to provide care defined by those who receive it" (Merryfeather & Bruce, 2014, p. 116).

LGBTQ PEOPLE AND CULTURAL COMPETENCE

The LGBTQ population is a global population that encompasses a wide intersectionality of people from many different communities and families. The current events in the global society are shaping and impacting the worldviews of people across the globe, which have direct implications to the care and understanding of LGBTQ populations. With that in mind, when nurses provide culturally competent care to LGBTQ people, they are in fact providing culturally competent nursing care to a wide breadth of diverse people.

For the nurse or provider to be culturally competent, they should

- ■ look inward at their own biases;
- ■ engage in educational activities that help to increase their knowledge of the LGBTQ population; and
  - ■ remedy their lack of knowledge about LGBTQ care to provide culturally competent care.

ASSESSING CULTURAL COMPETENCE IN NURSING CARE OF LGBTQ PEOPLE

To start the lifelong journey of cultural competence, first assess your own levels of cultural competence. This involves inward reflections on your own views and world understandings. This may be influenced by your past, upbringing, education, encounters with people, and a variety of variables.

Use the following statements and questions to explore your own individual cultural competence regarding LGBTQ people (see Exhibit 4.1). The purpose is to help you to consider your skills, knowledge, awareness, and attitude of yourself in your interactions with others. The goal is to help you to recognize what you can do to become more effective in caring for and interacting with LGBTQ people. Remember this is simply a tool and is not a test. The scale is there to help you identify areas of strength and areas that need further development in order to help you reach your goal of cultural competence.

Always remember that cultural competence is a process, and that learning occurs on a continuum and over a lifetime.

Fast Facts

Cultural competence in nursing practice focuses on knowledge, skill, attitude, and awareness. By consistently working toward being culturally competent, nurses are showing compassion and respect.

Exhibit 4.1

Individual LGBTQ Cultural Competence			
Knowledge	**Never**	**Sometimes**	**Always**
I will make mistakes and will learn from them.			
I understand that my knowledge of certain cultural groups is limited and commit seeking out opportunities to learn.			
I know that differences in gender identity and sexual orientation are important parts of an individuals identity that they value.			
I am knowledgeable about the history of the LGBTQ movement and the challenges faced by this population.			

Exhibit 4.1   *(continued)*

Individual LGBTQ Cultural Competence

Knowledge	Never	Sometimes	Always
I recognize that people have intersecting multiple identities drawn from race, sex, religion, ethnicity, and so forth and the importance of each of these identities varies from person to person.			
I recognize that stereotypical attitudes and discriminatory actions can dehumanize, even encourage violence against individuals because of their LGBTQ identity.			

Skill	Never	Sometimes	Always
I am developing skills to communicate effectively with individuals and groups.			
I am able to act in ways that demonstrate respect for the beliefs of others.			
I can recognize my own cultural biases in a given situation and I'm aware not to act out based on my biases			
I am learning about and able to put into practice practices which are necessary for my work—such as asking about gender identity, pronouns, and sexual orientation.			
My colleagues who are LGBTQ consider me an ally and know that I will support them.			

Exhibit 4.1   *(continued)*

Individual LGBTQ Cultural Competence

Awareness	Never	Sometimes	Always
I view differences as a positive.			
I have a clear sense of my own gender identity and sexual orientation.			
I am aware of the assumptions that I hold about LGBTQ people.			
I am aware of my discomfort when I encounter people have a different gender identity or sexual orientation than my own.			
I take any opportunity to put myself in places where I can learn about difference and create relationships.			
I am aware of how my cultural perspective influences my judgment about normal health behaviors and communication styles.			

Attitude	Never	Sometimes	Always
Male or female homosexuality or bisexuality is a natural expression of sexuality.			
A person who feels that their sex does not match their gender identity is wrong or confused.			

Exhibit 4.1 *(continued)*

Individual LGBTQ Cultural Competence

Attitude	Never	Sometimes	Always
Being transgender or gender nonbinary is a natural expression of gender identity.			
I would refuse to care for an LGBTQ patient.			
I feel that I would be able to talk to a patient who identifies as LGBTQ in a culturally appropriate manner.			
LGBTQ people have their own unique health needs and considerations for care that is important for nurses to know.			

Strategies and Tips to Grow Cultural Competence in Caring for LGBTQ People

- Reflect and complete a self-assessment of your own beliefs and values. How do these align with caring for LGBTQ people?
- Ask questions and take time to learn about what those answers mean to LGBTQ people.
- Use clear, descriptive communication that aligns with communication practices of your LGBTQ patient. Reflect the patient's language.
- Keep an open mind.
- Remember that it is impossible to ever become a true "expert."
- Expand and deepen your own LGBTQ knowledge base.
- Be aware of key LGBTQ terms and definitions.
- Create a welcoming environment for LGBTQ people.
- Use inclusive and gender-neutral language.
- Ask open-ended questions.
- Always convey dignity and respect.

Providing high-quality, culturally competent, patient-centered care to LGBTQ people requires ongoing learning and awareness. Knowledge building and gaining cultural competence among nurses must be viewed as opportunities rather than weaknesses. Nurses who have taken steps toward improving and understanding their cultural competency for LGBTQ patients can find new ways to address barriers to care and improve the health and well-being of LGBTQ people.

Further Reading

Carabez, R., Pellegrini, M., Mankovitz, A., Eliason, M., Ciano, M., & Scott, M. (2015). "Never in all my years...": Nurses' education about LGBT health. *Journal of Professional Nursing, 31*(4), 323–329. https://doi.org/10.1016/j.profnurs.2015.01.003

Carabez, R., Pellegrini, M., Mankovitz, A., Eliason, M., & Dariotis, W. (2014). Nursing students' perceptions of their knowledge of lesbian, gay, bisexual, and transgender issues: effectiveness of a multi-purpose assignment in a public health nursing class. *Journal of Nursing Education, 54*(1), 50–53. https://doi.org/10.3928/01484834-20141228-03

Fish, J., & Evans, D. (2016). Promoting cultural competency in nursing care of LGBT patients. *Journal of Research in Nursing, 21*(3), 159–162. https://doi.org/10.1177/1744987116643232

Gendron, T., Maddux, S., Krinsky, L., White, J., Lockeman, K., Metcalfe, Y., & Aggarwal, S. (2013). Cultural competence training for healthcare professionals working with LGBT older adults. *Educational Gerontology, 39*, 454–463. https://doi.org/10.1080/03601277.2012.701114

Lim, F., Brown, D., & Kim, S. (2014). Addressing health care disparities in the Lesbian, gay, bisexual, and transgender populations: a review of best practices. *The American Journal of Nursing, 114*(6), 24–34.

Lim, F., Johnson, M., & Eliason, M. (2015). A national survey of faculty knowledge, experience, and readiness for teaching lesbian, gay, bisexual, and transgender health in baccalaureate nursing programs. *Nursing Education Perspectives, 36*(4), 144–152.

Minority Health. (2021). *Think cultural health.* https://thinkculturalhealth.hhs.gov/

Moone, R., Croghan, C., & Olson, A. (2016). Why and how providers must build culturally competence, welcoming practices to serve LGBT elders. *Journal of the American Society on Aging, 40*(2), 73–77.

Traister, T. (2020). Improving LGBTQ cultural competence of RNs through education. *The Journal of Continuing Education in Nursing, 51*(8), 359–366. https://doi.org/10.3928/00220124-20200716-05

II

LGBTQ Health

5

Health Disparities of LGBTQ People

The LGBTQ population experience a higher prevalence of medical and behavioral issues. These issues are not unique to the LGBTQ population; instead, they were created and perpetuated by decades of discrimination and stigmatization in society and within healthcare. Nurses can better serve LGBTQ people to understand the health disparities that face this population. This will allow nurses to appropriately assess and educate LGBTQ people about their health and wellness.

In this chapter, you will learn:

1. The meaning of health disparities and social determinants of health
2. Health disparities faced by LGBTQ people
3. The nurse's role in reducing and eliminating health disparities

UNDERSTANDING DISPARITIES

Healthy People refer to the term *disparities* as a health outcome that is seen to a greater or lesser extent between populations (U.S. Department of Health and Human Services [HHS], 2020). Health disparities are often interpreted based on race or ethnicity; however, many dimensions can impact the degree of health disparities in the United States. Dimensions impacting health disparities are as follows:

- Race or ethnicity
- Sex

- Sexual identity
- Age
- Disability
- Socioeconomic status
- Geographic location

The health disparities of LGBTQ people are even more complicated because of a term called *intersectionality*. This term was coined by Kimberlé Crenshaw in 1991, who argued that people are marginalized by "discourses that are shaped to respond to one [identity] *or* the other," rather than both (Coleman, 2019).

For example, a lesbian has to deal with homophobia. A Black lesbian has to deal not only with homophobia but also with racism. This concept of intersectionality allows us to understand better the many facets of life and society that can impact the extent to which they experience health disparities. LGBTQ people's access to healthcare is affected by not only their gender identity or sexual orientation but also the dimensions previously mentioned.

The health disparities that face LGBTQ people are not unique to this population. They can be common clinical problems, such as smoking and obesity, or more nuanced like HIV infections, which require additional education and training.

Understanding the extent of health disparities faced by this population is challenging to estimate as there has historically not been national or state surveys that capture sexual orientation or gender identity information. In 2011, the Institute of Medicine released LGBT health that emphasized understanding LGBTQ health disparities and the collection of data to characterize LGBTQ health better.

When analyzing national data, there is limited to no domestic tracking or trending of the LGBT population. Collecting data among rare and stigmatized groups is a difficult undertaking as some LGBTQ people may fear retribution from answering research questions and polls. For example, LGBTQ people are not protected under many federal and state laws. With new religious protection laws, disclosure of their identity or orientation could lead to a loss of housing, employment, and even dire health implications. A Gallup Poll conducted in 2017 showed a record of 4.5% of Americans identified as LGBT (Newport, 2018). This was an increase from 4.1% in 2016 and 3.5% in 2012, the year that Gallup began tracking the measure. The data can show the population is either growing or people feel more comfortable identifying as LGBT in today's current society. As this number increases, we can expect nurses and healthcare providers to interact more frequently with LGBTQ people.

SOCIAL DETERMINANTS OF HEALTH

The driving forces in health disparities are the various social determinants of health of LGBTQ people. Social determinants of health care the conditions in which people are born, live, work, play, worship, and age. These conditions tremendously impact how people access healthcare, how they age and function, and their quality of life outcomes and risks.

Social determinates of health that impact LGBTQ people are primarily related to discrimination and oppression. Examples include:

- Lack of legislation protecting youth against bullying in schools
- Legal discrimination in denying access to healthcare, insurance, employment, housing, adoption, and retirement benefits
- Lack of social programs that are targeted to LGBTQ youth, adults, and senior citizens
- Healthcare systems that are not knowledgeable or culturally competent in LGBTQ health

Fast Facts

LGBTQ people have higher risks for suicide, homelessness, and certain cancers because of health disparities.

One way to understand how a health disparity forms is to look at when discrimination and stigma led to LGBTQ people using bars and clubs as a "safe place" (HHS, 2020). This, in part, has allowed alcohol abuse to normalize within this population. Research has shown that LGBTQ populations face higher rates of alcohol use than the general population.

Health Disparities of LGBTQ People

As mentioned earlier, the LGBTQ population encompasses a wide swath of people. Nurses must understand the different segments of the community also have various disparities. The examples from Table 5.1 can help to better understand the many different health disparities of LGBTQ people. When conducting a health assessment, nurses follow the role the social determinants of health can have with their patient's health and how being an LGBTQ person can impact their health.

Table 5.1

Summary of Health Disparities of LGBTQ Populations

LGBT youth	LGBT youth are two to three times more likely to attempt suicide. LGBT youth are more likely to be homeless.
Lesbians	Lesbians are less likely to get preventive services for cancer. Lesbians and bisexual females are more likely to be overweight or obese.
Gay men	Gay men are at higher risk of HIV and other STDs, especially among communities of color.
Transgender individuals	Transgender individuals have a high prevalence of: • HIV/STDs • Victimizations • Mental health issues • Suicide Transgender individuals are less likely to have health insurance than heterosexual or LGB individuals.
LGBT elderly	Elderly LGBT individuals face additional barriers to health because of isolation, lack of social services, and culturally competent providers.
LGBTQ populations	LGBT populations have the highest rates of tobacco, alcohol, and other drug use.

Source: Adapted from Healthy People 2020.

Note that although there are substantive reports on the existence of disparities faced by LGBTQ people, many in our country live healthy and productive lives. When interacting with patients, our assessments include their social support, socioeconomic status, and other determinants of health. This will allow the nurse and healthcare team to deliver patient-centered care.

CASE STUDY

A 23-year-old Black male named Jason, who is in graduate school, recently experienced an athletic injury. He is still having trouble with pain and goes to his healthcare provider for a follow-up appointment. During the intake assessment, the nurse, Meg, asks Jason about his alcohol consumption and drug use. Jason admits that he has been drinking more than usual because of the pain and that he has taken "some meds" from friends to help with his pain and to forget "other stuff."

Meg asks Jason further questions about "other stuff," and Jason reveals he has recently started having sex with men and women. He is worried that people might identify him as being gay and that his family and friends would find out and potentially ostracize him. Jason also discloses that since he has been having sex with men, he has developed anxious feelings about contracting HIV.

At this point in the conversation, Meg could do the following:

1. *Ignore Jason's discussion about his sexuality and remind him that he is here for pain management.*
2. *Let Jason know that the doctor will address all his concerns and talk about his sexuality with the doctor.*
3. *Respond in a culturally competent manner, which would be to validate Jason's experiences.*

Understanding the intersection of his many identities, such as a son, a friend, a student, an athlete, a bisexual, and a Black man, can help Meg to fully appreciate who Jason is as a person and how to best care for him. Meg should inform Jason his sexual preferences are real and that he should not be ashamed if he is bisexual, gay, or questioning. Knowing that Black men are at a higher risk of contracting HIV, Meg educates Jason about safe sex practices, such as condoms and PrEP.

Meg also informs Jason about LGBTQ resources that the practice offers and referral to specialty providers if he is ever interested in it. To wrap up the meeting before the provider comes in, Meg discusses the safety of taking pain medications, alcohol, and the consequences of misuse.

When interacting with LGBTQ patients, nurses and providers must affirm the normalcy and acceptance of their gender and sexual orientations. In doing so, the nurse is providing an opportunity to support the patient's engagement, which can improve health and mental health outcomes. During this scenario, it is also important not to reduce an LGBTQ person to or solely focus on their sexual behaviors. Understanding the intersectionality of identities (social, racial, economic, etc.) guides the nurse to approach the encounter and the person as a whole. This case study is an example of how nurses can create a culturally competent experience for an LGBTQ person to address and reduce health disparities.

Fast Facts

Nurses play a key role in addressing and reducing health disparities of LGBTQ people through culturally competent care.

Further Reading

Coleman, A. (2019, November 6). *What is intersectionality? A brief history of the theory.* https://time.com/5560575/intersectionality-theory/

Mayer, K. H., Potter, J., Goldhammer, H., & Makadon, H. J. (2015). *The Fenway guide to lesbian, gay, bisexual, and transgender health.* American College of Physicians.

Newport, F. (2018). *In U.S., estimate of LGBT population rises to 4.5%.* https://news.gallup.com/poll/234863/estimate-lgbt-population-rises.aspx

U.S. Department of Health and Human Services. (2020). *Lesbian, gay, bisexual, and transgender health.* https://www.healthypeople.gov/2020/topics-objectives/topic/lesbian-gay-bisexual-and-transgender-health

6

Stigma and Discrimination Against LGBTQ People

Stigma and discrimination are well-known barriers to culturally competent care for LGBTQ people. These forces work together to create personal, structural, and organizational barriers to accessing care. Stigma and discrimination are critical drivers in the health disparities of LGBTQ people. Nurses can help to decrease the health disparities faced by this vulnerable population by fighting discrimination and stigma. This chapter explores the concepts of stigma and discrimination and offers the nurse practical tips for improving access to inclusive care for LGBTQ people.

In this chapter, you will learn:

1. How stigma and discrimination impact LGBTQ patients
2. The concept of minority stress
3. How nurses can address stigma and discrimination in clinical settings

Stigma (negative and usually unfair beliefs) and discrimination (unfairly treating a person or group of people) against LGBTQ people can negatively affect this diverse population's health and well-being.

These negative beliefs and actions can affect the physical and mental health of LGBTQ and impact whether they seek and can get health services and the quality of the services they may receive. Such barriers to health must be addressed at different levels of society, such as healthcare settings, workplaces, and schools, to improve the health and well-being of LGBTQ people. Research suggests that LGBTQ individuals face health disparities linked to societal stigma, discrimination, such as higher rates of suicide, behavioral health concerns, and HIV.

Fast Facts

Stigma is the negative stereotype, and discrimination is the behavior that results from this negative stereotype.

STIGMA

Stigma often develops from a lack of understanding or fear. LGBTQ stigma refers to the intertwined social exclusion processes, devaluation, reduced access to opportunities, and power inequities impacting gender and sexual minorities (see Table 6.1). LGBTQ stigma, while a global phenomenon, is shaped by differences in history, geography, politics, culture, and media representation. Nurses may encounter the stigma of LGBTQ that depends on the location or area where they practice.

In healthcare, LGBTQ people have a history of stigmatization. Homosexuality was listed as a "sociopathic personality disorder" in the *Diagnostic and Statistical Manual of Psychological Disorders* (*DSM*) up until the 1970s. A transgender identity was also listed as a psychological disorder until 2013 in the *DSM*. This resulted in the pathologizing of sexual orientation and gender identities that fell outside of heterosexual and cisgender identities. As such, LGBTQ people were sometimes subject to traumatizing medical procedures

Table 6.1

Three Types of Stigma	
Stigma	**Description**
Public stigma	Negative or discriminatory attitudes others have about mental illness.
Self-stigma	Negative attitudes, including internalized shame, that people with mental illness have about their condition.
Institutional stigma	More systemic, involving government and private organizations that intentionally or unintentionally limit opportunities for people with mental illness. Examples include lower funding for mental illness research or fewer mental health services relative to other healthcare.

Source: American Psychiatric Association. (2020). *Stigma and discrimination*. https://www.psychiatry.org/patients-families/stigma-and-discrimination

and interventions, such as conversion therapy, castrations, and electroshock (Barrett & Wholihan, 2016).

DISCRIMINATION

In some places, discrimination and abuse may not be as overt, but it exists nonetheless. Most LGBTQ people have encountered prejudice and bias throughout their lives, and these experiences play a role in how they interact with the healthcare system (see Box 6.1). For older LGBTQ adults, this is especially true as they came of age when discrimination was much more commonplace and a part of our laws, policies, and healthcare educations.

Although today's landscape appears much more welcoming for LGBTQ people, many still report various forms of discrimination.

Fast Facts

Discrimination is an almost universal experience among LGBTQ people, with upward of 90% believing that it exists and many who have experienced it.

Discrimination Statistics for LGBTQ

- 90% of all LGBTQ people believe there is discrimination against gay, lesbian, and bisexual people in America today.
- 91% of all LGBTQ people believe there is discrimination against transgender and gender nonconforming people.
- 33% say the bigger problem is discrimination based on laws and government policies.

Percentage of LGBTQ Americans saying they (or an LGBTQ friend or family member) have experienced the following forms of discrimination because they are LGBTQ:

- 57% threats or nonsexual harassment
- 51% sexual harassment
- 51% violence
- 34% verbal harassment of questioning in a bathroom

Source: NPR/Robert Wood Johnson Foundation/Harvard T.H. Chan School of Public Health, Discrimination in America: Experiences and Views of LGBTQ Americans, January 26–April 9, 2017. Q93a/b/e, Q94. Each question asked of half-sample. Total (*N*) = 489 LGBTQ U.S. adults.

BOX 6.1 TRANSGENDER EXPERIENCES IN HEALTHCARE

- 29% said a doctor or other healthcare provider refused to see them because of their actual or perceived gender identity.
- 12% said a doctor or other healthcare provider refused to give them healthcare related to gender transition.
- 23% said a doctor or other healthcare provider intentionally misgendered them or used the wrong name.
- 21% said a doctor or other healthcare provider used harsh or abusive language when treating them.
- 29% said they experienced unwanted physical contact from a doctor or other healthcare provider (such as fondling, sexual assault, or rape).

Source: Mirza, S. A., & Rooney, C. (2019, August 13). *Discrimination prevents LGBTQ people from accessing health care*. https://www.americanprogress.org/issues/lgbtq-rights/news/2018/01/18/445130/discrimination-prevents-lgbtq-people-accessing-health-care/

These statistics are vital to nurses because they show the extent of discrimination faced by the LGBTQ population. LGBTQ patients who have experienced discrimination because of their identity may fear coming out to their nurse or healthcare provider because of previous discrimination they have faced. For some, even though they have not been personally discriminated against, because they know this data or know of someone who has had that experience, they may delay or not seek out healthcare.

CASE STUDY: BOBBI AND MATTEA

Bobbi is a 34-year-old female who arrives in the ED. Bobbi was brought to the ED by her girlfriend Mattea. Bobbi and Mattea were assaulted by a group of people who saw them holding hands and repeatedly yelled slurs at the couple. Bobbi has multiple contusions and abrasions and is worried that she may have a broken rib. The nurse notices that Mattea is very protective of Bobbi and appears distrustful of the nursing staff.

In this scenario, it is possible that both Bobbi and Mattea are apprehensive and scared of how they will be treated in the hospital. After being attacked for their sexual orientation, they might wonder:

- *"How will the nurse respond?"*
- *"Will they think I deserved this?"*
- *"Will they treat my injuries?"*

Nursing staff must welcome both Bobbi and Mattea by validating their experiences, ensuring that it is communicated that they are safe in their hospital, and communicate clearly about the care they will receive and the next steps.

MINORITY STRESS

The health issues that LGBT people experience are often exacerbated by the discrimination they face in society. A range of harms is related to "minority stress," or the added stressors individuals face because they belong to a stigmatized group. Minority stress has widespread research support in explaining health disparities experienced by sexual and gender minorities. Minority stress can be understood as "minority groups experience stress stemming from experiences of stigma and discrimination." LGBT people experience forms of minority stress shared with other marginalized groups, such as discrimination, the expectation of rejection and prejudice-related life events (e.g., hate crimes), as well as unique stressors such as identity concealment and internalized homophobia (McConnell et al., 2018).

Fast Facts

Minority stress can also impact LGBTQ people who have never personally been discriminated against. As a collective group, the individual knows that this discrimination exists, so they, in turn, expect the bias to happen to them.

For nurses, this is a critical concept when we encounter LGBTQ people in the clinical setting; we use this understanding of minority stress to guide the nurse–patient relationship. Realizing that the patient expects to be discriminated against can allow us to optimize care by communicating effectively, validating their concerns, and delivering culturally competent care to this vulnerable population. In doing so, nurses play a crucial role in breaking the cycle of minority stress and positively impacting the health and well-being of LGBTQ people.

HOW NURSES CAN COMBAT DISCRIMINATION AND STIGMA

- Create a welcoming environment that is inclusive of LGBTQ patients.
  - Prominently post nondiscrimination policies in clinical settings.
  - Display LGBTQ-friendly symbols on staff badges, placards, and waiting areas.
  - Create or designate unisex or single-stall restrooms.
- Foster an environment that supports and nurtures all patients and families.
  - Refrain from assuming a person's sexual or gender identity.
  - Be aware of misconceptions, biases, and stereotypes.
  - Ensure that clinical staff treat all patients with dignity and respect.
- Advocate for inclusive forms and allow for self-identification of sexual orientation and gender identity.
- Advocate for policies and legislation supporting equal access to high-quality, culturally congruent healthcare for LGBTQ+ populations.
- Promote research and interventions aimed at improving the health, wellness, and needs of LGBTQ+ populations.
- Incorporate the issues of the LGBTQ+ populations as part of the nursing curriculum.
- Support for nurses and other healthcare providers who are bullied or witness others being bullied or discriminated against.

CASE STUDY

Kel is currently in the 9th grade and is starting to identify as a transgender male. Kel's assigned sex at birth was female, and his birth name was Kelli. He has just recently began outwardly showing his male identity and gender expression. Kel arrives to the school nurse appearing to be in acute distress, anxious, tearful, and stuttering their words. After a few moments, Kel is able to tell the school nurse that he was kicked out of the boy's bathroom by one of the teachers. While leaving the bathroom, several students called Kel a freak and not knowing what to do, he came to the nurse's office.

1. *How can the school nurse best support Kel in this immediate situation?*
   a. *The school nurse should recognize that Kel is experiencing distress from the trauma of being removed from the bathroom and bullied by his peers and also the stress of understanding and navigating their own internal gender identity and sense of self. The school nurse should validate Kel's feelings and provide him with an outlet for this distress.*

   b. *The school nurse should assess Kel for immediate harm or injury—does he need to go to the ED? Should the nurse call his parents to take him home? Does Kel need to see a therapist or counselor if one is available at the school? School nurses interacting may be the first to notice when students present with behavioral health concerns from experiences with discrimination family rejection related to their gender identity. School nurses can often be the first people to provide intervention, referrals, and resources.*

2. *How can the school nurse best support Kel and other transgender or gender nonbinary students?*

   a. *There are many resources available to assist the school nurse with learning more about transgender and gender nonbinary youth. This learning is important because it can help the nurse to better understand and validate Kel's experiences and existence.*

   b. *Given that the social recognition and use of a transgender student's preferred name is associated with lower depression, suicidal ideation, and suicidal behaviors, it is important that the school nurse advocate for the school to use a student's preferred name and to always use this name when interacting with students.*

   c. *Pronoun use has an enormous impact on the transgender student's mental health. By being a model for the school staff, the school nurse's actions of respecting a student's preferred pronoun may inspire others to do the same.*

   d. *The school nurse's bathroom can be offered as a private place for the students to use to alleviate their discomfort in being in the locker rooms—whether they are cisgender or transgender. The school nurse should be proactive in making that option known to all students.*

3. *What actions can the nurse do in the school or work setting to help combat stigma and discrimination?*

   a. *A simple intervention to combat discrimination or bullying is by displaying signs of being a transgender ally in visible locations.*

   b. *Nurses are well positioned to foster an accepting environment that confronts erroneous notions that contribute to fear-based beliefs.*

   c. *The school nurse can provide evidence-based education to the staff, school board, and other students about gender identity sexual orientation. Providing this education can play a key role in reducing the stigma and discrimination that transgender and other LGBTQ students may experience.*

Fast Facts

Nurses are well equipped to address stigma and discrimination in healthcare and creating inclusive care environments.

Further Reading

American Psychiatric Association. (2020). *Stigma and discrimination*. https://www.psychiatry.org/patients-families/stigma-and-discrimination

Barrett, N., & Wholihan, D. (2016). Providing palliative care to LGBTQ patients. *Nursing Clinics of North America, 51*(3), 501–511. https://doi.org/10.1016/j.cnur.2016.05.001

Casey, L. S., Reisner, S. L., Findling, M. G., Blendon, R. J., Benson, J. M., Sayde, J. M., & Miller, C. (2019). Discrimination in the United States: Experiences of lesbian, gay, bisexual, transgender, and queer Americans. *Health Services Research, 54*(Suppl. 2), 1454–1466. https://doi.org/10.1111/1475-6773.13229

Centers for Disease Control and Prevention. (2016, February 29). *Stigma and discrimination affects gay and bisexual men's health*. https://www.cdc.gov/msmhealth/stigma-and-discrimination.htm

Healthy People 2030. (n.d.). *LGBT*. Retrieved January 29, 2021, from https://health.gov/healthypeople/objectives-and-data/browse-objectives/lgbt

Mattocks, K. M., Sullivan, J. C., Bertrand, C., Kinney, R. L., Sherman, M. D., & Gustason, C. (2015). Perceived stigma, discrimination, and disclosure of sexual orientation among a sample of lesbian veterans receiving care in the department of veterans affairs. *LGBT Health, 2*(2), 147–153. https://doi.org/10.1089/LGBT.2014.0131

McConnell, E. A., Janulis, P., Phillips, G., 2nd, Truong, R., & Birkett, M. (2018). Multiple minority stress and LGBT community resilience among sexual minority men. *Psychology of Sexual Orientation and Gender Diversity, 5*(1), 1–12. https://doi.org/10.1037/sgd0000265

Menkin, D., & Flores, D. D. (2019). Transgender students: Advocacy, care, and support opportunities for school nurses. *NASN School Nurse, 34*(3), 173–177. https://doi.org/10.1177/1942602X18801938

MinorityHealth. (n.d.). *Think cultural health*. Retrieved January 29, 2021, from https://thinkculturalhealth.hhs.gov/

Mirza, S. A., & Rooney, C. (2019, August 13). *Discrimination prevents LGBTQ people from accessing health care*. https://www.americanprogress.org/issues/lgbtq-rights/news/2018/01/18/445130/discrimination-prevents-lgbtq-people-accessing-health-care/

Stangl, A. L., Earnshaw, V. A., Logie, C. H., van Brakel, W., Simbayi, L. C., Barré, I., & Dovidio, J. F.. (2019). The health stigma and discrimination framework: A global, crosscutting framework to inform research, intervention development, and policy on health-related stigmas. *BMC Medicine, 17*, 31. https://doi.org/10.1186/s12916-019-1271-3

7

LGBTQ Substance Use and Substance Use Disorders

Substance use disorders and misuse carry their stereotypes and stigma that can be compounded within the LGBTQ community. This chapter explores the difference between substance use and substance use disorder, commonly used substances, and the role of the nurse in helping LGBTQ patients navigate substance use to improve overall well-being.

In this chapter, you will learn:

1. The prevalence of substance use disorders in LGBTQ populations
2. Common substance abuse disorders experienced by LGBTQ people and various substances that are misused by this community
3. Screening techniques and treatment strategies that nurses can incorporate into clinical practice

SUBSTANCE ABUSE IN LGBTQ INDIVIDUALS

Research on substance use in the LGBTQ community did not start until around the 1970s. Even in the present day, there is not much data on transgender people. Evidence is also lacking in the recovery outcomes of LGBTQ people or how they compare to heterosexual people. Recently, federally funded surveys have started to include sexual orientation and gender identity identification questions in

Table 7.1

Substance Use Facts	
All drug use	LGBTQ are more than twice as likely as heterosexual adults (39.1% vs. 17.1%) to have used any illicit drug in the past year.
Marijuana	A third of sexual minority adults (30.7%) used marijuana in the past year, compared to 12.9% of heterosexual adults.
Prescription pain relievers	1 in 10 (10.4%) misused prescription pain relievers, compared to 4.5% of heterosexual adults.
Alcohol	Higher percentage of LGBT adults between 18 and 64 reported past-year binge drinking (five or more drinks on a single occasion) than heterosexual adults.

Source: National Institute on Drug Abuse. (2020, August 25). *Substance use and suds in LGBTQ* populations*. https://www.drugabuse.gov/drug-topics/substance-use-suds-in-lgbtq-populations

their research. From this, studies have found that LGBTQ people have higher rates of substance misuse and substance use disorders (Table 7.1 and Figures 7.1 and 7.2).

Some LGBTQ people have used alcohol and other substances to cope with various forms of stigma and discrimination. Some may use substances to deal with prior to coming out to family and friends. This coping mechanism could be a fear of unsupportive families, religion, and relationships in their lives. Alcohol and other substances can also be used to decrease inhibitions and less anxiety in social and sexual encounters.

Fast Facts

Some LGBTQ people use substances to medicate because of their minority status.

Common acts of drinking alcohol and cigarette smoking may have led to the socialization and acceptance of these behaviors within this community. Previously, it was mentioned how LGBTQ people used bars and clubs as a safe place to meet people and find sexual or romantic partners. This broader acceptance of substance use behaviors may place LGBTQ people at risk of exposure to addictive substances through various social networks. LGBTQ and drug use can also be associated with the "club scene," where people utilize multiple drugs such as alcohol, alkyl nitrites (poppers), cocaine, ketamine, and others.

Fast Facts

LGBTQ people have higher rates of substance use than heterosexual individuals.

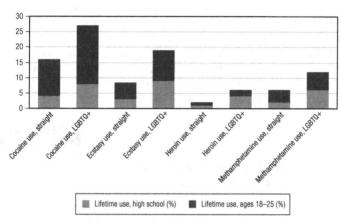

Figure 7.1 Sexual identity and lifetime hard drug use.

Source: Data from Trevor Project. (2020, March 26). *Research brief: Substance use disparities by sexual identity*. https://www.thetrevorproject.org/2020/03/26/research-brief-substance-use-disparities-by-sexual-identity

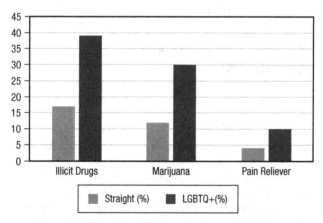

Figure 7.2 Substance abuse rates among LGBTQ community compared to straight community.

Source: Data from Mission Harbor Behavioral Health. (2021). *LGBTQ Friendly Rehab and Mental Health Treatment Center guide*. https://sbtreatment.com/resources/lgbtq-friendly-guide

Providers and nurses who are working with LGBTQ people with addictions and those in recovery have to understand the depth of psychosocial and cultural aspects of the individual's addiction. Depending on the LGBTQ person's social network, substances can be ever-present, leaving individuals with few events considered sober. Those with a history of addiction and in recovery, triggers, and cues can be ever-present. Are they abusing alcohol because they have a fear of coming out? Are they engaging in illicit drug use to reduce inhibitions to engage in sexual activity? Nurses caring for these individuals must examine the intersection of the person's addiction and/or recovery. This could be by helping them address internalized homophobia or transphobia or by helping someone develop a social network that is not centered around bars or clubs.

Fast Facts

Be careful not to automatically attribute LGBTQ patients' substance use to their sexual and/or gender identity.

Although their sexual and/or gender identity can play a role for some, LGBTQ people use substances for many of the same reasons as their heterosexual counterparts. It is important to note the majority of the LGBTQ population in the United States and globally do not use substances. For many of those who do engage in substance use, they can use it without any associated harm (Abdulrahim et al., 2016).

SUBSTANCE ABUSE, DEPENDENCE, AND USE DISORDERS—EXPLAINED

- Substance use exists on a spectrum that ranges from abstinence to addiction.
- Substance abuse is a *pattern of substance use leading to significant impairment or distress and impacts a significant role obligation (such as school, work, home), involves situations that are physically hazardous (driving), frequent legal problems, and/or continued use despite social or interpersonal issues* over 12 months.
- Substance dependence is a *maladaptive pattern of use leading to significant impairment or distress and impacts three or more of the following within the same 12-month period*—tolerance markedly increased that the individual consumes more substance to achieve same intoxication level, withdrawal symptoms or use of substances

BOX 7.1 THE *DSM 5* OUTLINES 10 DIFFERENT CLASSES OF DRUGS THAT A DIAGNOSIS OF SUBSTANCE USE DISORDER CAN BE APPLIED

- Alcohol
- Caffeine
- Cannabis
- Hallucinogens (phencyclidine and other hallucinogens, such as LSD)
- Inhalants
- Opioids
- Sedatives (including hypnotics or anxiolytics)
- Stimulants
- Tobacco
- Other (or unknown)

to avoid withdrawal, a more substantial amount of substances or a more extended period abused, persistent or unsuccessful attempts to control substance use.

- In the *DSM 5*, the diagnosis of a substance abuse disorder is based on a pathological pattern of behaviors related to substance use (Box 7.1). An essential characteristic of substance use disorders is an underlying change in brain circuits that may persist beyond detoxification. Substance use disorders are diagnosed by a mental health professional.

Commonly Used Substances

This section will provide the reader with a basic overview of common substances and the effects that they produce. For more information, consult with an addiction medicine specialist.

Fast Facts

Alcohol, tobacco, and marijuana use is normative in the United States. Substance use disorders are a pattern of substance use over a substantial period that causes biological (withdrawal, tolerance, craving), interpersonal/social, or workplace problems that invoke stress.

ALCOHOL

Alcohol is one of the oldest and most widely used substances. This substance is legally available in the United States and most parts globally. Easily accessible and socially embedded in many interactions.

Hepatotoxic—leading cause of cirrhosis worldwide, special considerations for patients to avoid medications containing acetaminophen

Intoxication symptoms:

- Decreased anxiety
- Memory and coordination impairments
- Lowers respiratory system function

Withdrawal symptoms:

- Increased anxiety and/or heart rate
- Tremors
- Risk of seizure

Fast Facts

Alcohol withdrawal can be lethal, and detoxification should be completed under medical supervision. Withdrawal symptoms can begin up to 72 hours after the last alcohol use.

GAMMA-HYDROXYBUTYRATE

This substance is commonly considered a "club drug." GHB is a naturally occurring neurotransmitter in the body. This substance is legally prescribed to treat narcolepsy and is available in different forms, such as its precursor gamma-butyrolactone. Some LGBTQ people abuse this drug to obtain muscle mass. This drug is also commonly abused at circuit parties to help decrease inhibitions and improve sexual experiences.

Intoxication symptoms:

- Euphoria
- Dizziness
- Overdose
- Coma

Withdrawal symptoms:

- Increased anxiety and heart rate
- Tremors
- Carries a risk of seizures

OPIATE AND OPIOID NARCOTICS

Medically indicated to treat pain, cough suppression, and/or as an antidiarrheal. Many forms of this class exist—natural opiates (morphine), semisynthetic (codeine and heroin), and synthetic (hydrocodone, oxycodone, etc.).

Intoxication symptoms:

- Euphoria
- Analgesia
- Sedation
- Constricted pupils
- Constipation

Withdrawal symptoms:

- Increased gastrointestinal motility
- Diarrhea
- Nausea
- Piloerection (goosebumps)

Injected opiates, such as heroin, have a higher risk of contracting HIV and hepatitis B and C. Some data has shown that LGBTQ people use injectable opiates at a lower rate than the general population but use prescription at similar levels.

MARIJUANA

The cannabis plant can be smoked or eaten as an intoxicant. Many states in the United States have made legalized the use of recreational and medicinal marijuana consumption. There are no formal guidelines for medical marijuana, but it can be used for reducing nausea and vomiting, increasing appetite, decreasing chronic pain, seizure control, and anxiety disorders.

Intoxication symptoms:

- Euphoria
- Relaxation

- Increased sensory experiences
- Delayed reaction time

Withdrawal symptoms:

- Only seen with heavy and regular use
- Insomnia
- Irritability

COCAINE

A stimulant made from the leaves of the coca plant. Cocaine can be injected but is most commonly snorted in powder form. Crack is a form of freebased cocaine that is smoked in a glass pipe and inhaled.

Cardiotoxic—long-term use can lead to arrhythmias and myocardial infarctions

Intoxication symptoms:

- Increased heart rate euphoria
- Disinhibition
- Increased anxiety
- Paranoia
- Hallucinations

Withdrawal symptoms:

- Fatigue
- Depressed mood

AMPHETAMINE-TYPE STIMULANTS

Amphetamine, methamphetamine, and several related drugs are all synthetic stimulants that impact dopamine receptors. Similar to cocaine, they are a stimulant but usually last much longer. These stimulants can be ingested, snorted, smoked, and some even inserted anally.

These medications can be prescribed legally for use in narcolepsy or attention deficit hyperactivity disorder (ADHD).

Intoxication symptoms:

- Increased heart rate euphoria
- Disinhibition
- Increased anxiety
- Paranoia
- Hallucinations

Withdrawal symptoms:

- Fatigue
- Depressed mood

Other substances that can be seen misused in the LGBTQ community include hallucinogens (commonly ketamine), alkyl nitrites (poppers), and pro-erectile drugs. See Table 7.2.

TREATMENT AND INTERVENTIONS

Screening

The screening of patients is essential in all care settings. Intake and patient assessments should include questions about substance use. Normalizing questions about substance use in health assessments can help to create open communication and allow patients to feel that they are not being singled out for their use history. There are many screening tools available to nurses and providers interested in incorporating them into their assessments. Polysubstance use is common—if a person is having problems with one substance, they are likely using and may be having problems with other substances. Nurses and other providers must screen for and treat all substance use disorders and problem substance use.

Table 7.2

LGBTQ Slang for Common Drugs	
Slang	Definition
Crystal, tina	Methamphetamine
Cri-cri	Spanish term for methamphetamine
K-hole	Ketamine blackout
Booty bump	Use of methamphetamine or other substance, administered rectally for faster absorption
Tina and her evil sister	Tina = methamphetamine Evil sister = ketamine
420, 4:20, 4:20	Marijuana or marijuana friendly
Tweaked/tweaking	High on stimulants
Rush, jungle juice	Nitrite inhalants (poppers)
Party and play or PnP	Use of methamphetamine or other drugs during sex

Brief Interventions

This method of intervening often works with alcohol use and cigarette smoking. Healthcare providers identify hazardous substance use and attempt a "brief intervention." Here is an example.

1. Ask the patient about their smoking habits.
2. Advise the patient your professional opinion is that they quit smoking now or in the next 30 days.
3. Assess if the patient is willing to quit.
4. Assist the patient by providing interventions such as education, referrals, and other resources.
5. Arrange follow-up and support.

Treatments

Pharmacotherapies—available for the treatment of alcohol, nicotine, and opioid dependence.

Behavioral therapies—cognitive behavioral therapy (CBT), motivational interviewing, and contingency management.

Substance use is not unique to the LGBTQ community, but it can present challenges because of the health disparities faced by this population. Not all LGBTQ people who use substances will need treatment, but some will. Be prepared to assess and support their LGBTQ patients for substance use and understand that mental health and trauma can play a role in the development of substance use problems. Culturally competent care of this population will help the nurse and medical team to tailor treatment and interventions to improve health outcomes.

CASE STUDY BY CRAIG RICCELLI, MD

Misty is a 19-year-old cisgender female who presents to the ED seeking detoxification from daily opioid use. Misty reports to the psychiatric nurse that she has been using heroin daily for the last several months and that she is experiencing homelessness. She states she was kicked out of her parents' home approximately 1 year ago after disclosing that she identifies as a lesbian. She moved in with her significant other. However, she is also using heroin daily. They were evicted from the apartment several weeks ago due to finances. When mentioning her significant other, Misty shifts her eye contact to the floor and appears distressed.

1. *What additional substance use history is important for the psychiatric nurse to obtain?*
   a. *Ask about benzodiazepines and alcohol use. Both of these can be associated with life-threatening withdrawal.*
   b. *Inquire about the route in which Misty is using heroin as intravenous use is a significant risk factor for infectious diseases such as hepatitis C and HIV.*
   c. *When did Misty begin struggling with substance use? LGBTQ-specific sociocultural influences often contribute to the development of substance use disorders among LGBTQ young adults.*
2. *What additional social history is important to obtain?*
   a. *The nurse should screen for trauma through a trauma-informed care approach. LGBTQ patients are at increased risk for experiencing trauma especially in the transitional age. Post-traumatic stress disorder includes symptoms of avoidance, which can manifest as substance use. If she is experiencing abuse from her significant other, her safety may be in jeopardy.*
3. *What resources and psychoeducation should the nurse recommend and provide to Misty?*
   a. *Evidence suggests that opioid use disorders are disproportionately prevalent in the LGBTQ community. Programs that integrate behavioral health with primary care, address minority stress, and use a trauma-informed approach have the most potential to produce effective, long-term benefits for LGBTQ people with opioid use disorders. Some faith-based resources may discriminate against LGBTQ and cause additional stress. It is important for the nurse to have an understanding of community resources that are appropriate and accepting of LGBTQ people.*
   b. *Psychoeducation should focus on identifying ways of socializing outside of substance-saturated environments.*

Fast Facts

Effective treatments for substance use disorders exist and include behavioral therapies. LGBTQ people should be screened and supported to ensure success.

Further Reading

Abdulrahim, D., Whiteley, C., Moncrieff, M., & Bowden-Jones, O. (2016). *Club drug use among lesbian, gay, bisexual and trans (LGBT) people.* Novel Psychoactive Treatment UK Network (NEPTUNE).

American Psychiatric Association. (2013). *Diagnostic and statistical manual of mental disorders* (5th ed.). https://doi.org/10.1176/appi.books.978 0890425596

HealthyPeople.gov. (n.d.). *Lesbian, gay, bisexual, and transgender health.* Retrieved January 17, 2021, from https://www.healthypeople.gov/2020/topics-objectives/topic/lesbian-gay-bisexual-and-transgender-health

Mayer, K. H., Potter, J., Goldhammer, H., & Makadon, H. J. (2015). *The Fenway guide to lesbian, gay, bisexual, and transgender health.* American College of Physicians.

Mission Harbor Behavioral Health. (2021). *LGBTQ Friendly Rehab and Mental Health Treatment Center guide.* https://sbtreatment.com/resources/lgbtq-friendly-guide/

National Institute on Drug Abuse. (2020, August 25). *Substance use and suds in LGBTQ* populations.* https://www.drugabuse.gov/drug-topics/substance-use-suds-in-lgbtq-populations

SAMHSA. (2020). *2019 National survey on drug use and health: Lesbian, gay, & bisexual (LGB) adults: CBHSQ data.* https://www.samhsa.gov/data/report/2019-nsduh-lesbian-gay-bisexual-lgb-adults

Trevor Project. (2020, March 26). *Research brief: Substance use disparities by sexual identity.* https://www.thetrevorproject.org/2020/03/26/research-brief-substance-use-disparities-by-sexual-identity/

8

LGBTQ Behavioral Health

This chapter will explore the behavioral health of LGBTQ people and the challenges that they may face. The nurse will learn how stigma and discrimination toward LGBTQ people can create serious mental health consequences. The chapter will explore mental health in relation to LGBTQ people and use case examples to highlight key points.

In this chapter, you will learn:

1. The background of how healthcare approached LGBTQ people
2. General considerations and key understandings of LGBTQ behavioral health
3. How the nurse can conduct a culturally competent and sensitive mental health assessment

BACKGROUND OF LGBTQ MENTAL HEALTH

Healthcare in the United States and globally has a history of associating LGBTQ identities with mental illness and abnormalities. Early psychiatric theory and psychologists linked homosexuality and gender nonconformity as pathologic in nature and claimed it could be "cured" or "repaired." It was not until 1973 that the American Psychiatric Association removed the diagnosis of homosexuality from the *Diagnostic and Statistical Manual of Mental Disorders (DSM)*, Second Edition, and all major professional behavioral health groups have since made statements to affirm that homosexuality is not a mental disorder. Gender dysphoria is currently listed in the *DSM-5*. Some argue that this inclusion of gender dysphoria as a diagnosis pathologizes the identities of transgender people; however, others believe this inclusion in the *DSM* provides access to medical treatment (such as hormones and gender-affirming surgeries).

Stigma and Discrimination

Many of the behavioral health concerns that are faced by LGBTQ people are similar to those of the general population. Some LGBTQ people, however, may present with behavioral health concerns that are specific to their sexual or gender identity. A common experience to LGBTQ people is individual and systemic oppression as a result of stigma and discrimination.

Stigma and discrimination based on sexual orientation and/or gender identity have negative impacts on the mental health of LGBTQ people. LGBTQ people may face bullying, reduced family acceptance, and sexual and physical assault. All of which are risk factors for behavioral health issues.

Fast Facts

The stress caused by stigma and discrimination can negatively impact the behavioral health of LGBTQ people.

Mental Health Disparities

- LGBTQ individuals are more than twice as likely as heterosexual men and women to have a mental health disorder in their lifetime.
- LGBTQ individuals are 2.5 times more likely to experience depression, anxiety, and substance misuse compared with heterosexual individuals.
- LGBTQ individuals have higher rates of mental health service use than their heterosexual counterparts.

LGBTQ MENTAL HEALTH: CONSIDERATIONS FOR NURSES

Coming Out

- A process in which an LGBTQ person accepts and discloses their sexual orientation or gender identity.
- This process can be lifelong for some people and is often nonlinear.
  - For example, a person who is out at their current job or situation (friends, family, etc.) may have to repeat this process at new jobs, events, and scenarios.
  - In the clinical setting, LGBTQ people may be hesitant to "come out" to a nurse or provider. For each clinical encounter with nursing staff—new admissions, change of shift, and so forth—the patient must continuously come out.
- The nurse may help someone with the coming out process as follows:
  - By providing support and assessing the patient's coping and support systems.
    - By assisting in finding community supports, such as therapy, housing, and support groups.
  - By helping the patient see the positive aspects of coming out.
    - They no longer have to hide a major part of their life and identity from family and friends.
    - Self-acceptance can help them lead a more fulfilling and authentic life and shift from shame-based thinking.

Rejection

- Coming out can be a traumatic or difficult experience for some LGBTQ people (see Box 8.1).
  - Coping with rejection can lead to behavioral health concerns and maladaptive coping mechanisms.

BOX 8.1 COMING OUT AS LGBTQ

A GLAAD poll conducted in 2018 showed people's discomfort about learning that a family member is LGBTQ:

> 36% of people aged 18 to 34
> 30% of people aged 35 to 51
> 29% of people aged 52 to 71
> 34% of people aged 72+

Source: Miller, S. (2019, June 24). The young are regarded as the most tolerant generation. That's why results of this LGBTQ survey are `alarming.' https://www.usatoday.com/story/news/nation/2019/06/24/lgbtq-acceptance-millennials-decline-glaad-survey/1503758001/

- Rejection can lead to feelings of guilt, shame, and fears about physical safety.
- LGBTQ youth who have rejecting families are more eight times more likely to attempt suicide and having at least one supportive adult in their lives reduces that risk by 40%.

Aging

- Older adults of today's generation have lived through many defining moments of LGBTQ history and likely experienced discrimination:
  - The birth of the modern-day rights movement of Stonewall.
  - The AIDS epidemic.
  - Various federal and state legislation forbidding or outlawing their sexual orientation and gender identity.
- Older LGBTQ adults may be less trustful of healthcare providers and less likely to disclose their sexual orientation or gender identity.
- Aging gay men may feel isolated or lonely as gay male culture places an emphasis on the value of youth and physical beauty.
- Bisexual seniors report higher rates of depression, anxiety and suicidal ideation than their gay and lesbian counterparts.
- LGBTQ older adults face a number of unique challenges, including the combination of anti-LGBTQ stigma and ageism. Approximately 31% of LGBTQ older adults report depressive symptoms; 39% report serious thoughts of taking their own lives.
- Nurses can create a therapeutic relationship with the patient through open communication.
  - For some patients, acknowledging the past and how homophobia and discrimination have impacted their lives can create a meaningful and lasting impact.
  - Explore social support and social networks as these could play a role in decreased health outcomes.

Fast Facts

Nurses who work with LGBTQ people should provide them with care and communication that validates and affirms their identities.

Dual Stigma

- A phenomenon when an individual with a behavioral health concern or psychiatric diagnosis is a member of a stigmatized group.
- Can also be referred to as a *double stigma.*
- LGBTQ people must navigate the stigma, prejudice, and discrimination surrounding their sexual orientation or gender identity in addition to the bias against mental illness.
- Nurses must be aware of the multiple existences that their patients experience within their lives such as race, gender, ethnicity, and socioeconomic status. Better understanding the patient's experience with these factors will enable the nurse to validate their existence with multiple stigmas and help create an environment of inclusion and acceptance.

Fast Facts

LGBTQ people with a behavioral health diagnosis have to manage both the stigma of being LGBTQ as well as the stigma of mental illnesses.

Trauma

- LGBTQ may experience trauma as a result of their sexual orientation or gender identity.
  - Types of trauma may include:
    - Labeling
    - Stereotyping
    - Denial of access to care
    - Verbal, mental, and physical abuse
    - Purposeful misgendering
  - The LGBTQ population is one of the most targeted communities for hate crimes in the United States (National Alliance on Mental Illness [NAMI], 2020).
- Trauma experienced by an individual can lead to a heightened risk of posttraumatic stress disorder (PTSD).
- Understand an LGBTQ person's risk for trauma is important to nurses and other healthcare providers.

CASE EXAMPLE

Max arrives to the ED with his partner after being assaulted. Max and his partner report that they were holding hands walking down the street when they were attacked by a person who yelled gay slurs at them and then assaulted him. Max appears fearful and apprehensive in speaking with the nurse in the examination room. When the nurse goes to assess Max, he flinches away.

In this scenario, it is crucial that the nurse communicates with caring and cultural competence. Max, who was just assaulted, might be fearful that the nurse and healthcare team will treat him differently. Max might worry that the nurses or doctor will think he "deserved" the assault or that they might treat him with less compassion because he is a gay man.

When someone like Max is attacked for the sexual orientation or gender identity, it can lead further stress on future encounters, regardless of the nurse's intentions. The nurse's role is to validate their experience, condemn discrimination, and care for people like Max with dignity and respect.

Substance Misuse

- Substance overuse or misuse may be used by LGBTQ as a coping mechanism or a method of self-medication.
- LGBTQ people face higher rates of substance use disorders than the general population.
- Research has shown that treatment programs that specialize in treating LGBTQ people have better outcomes when LGBTQ people participate compared to general programs (NAMI, 2020).
- Women who identify as lesbian/bisexual are more than twice as likely to engage in heavy (alcohol) drinking in the past month than heterosexual women (8.0% vs. 4.4%).
- Gay/bisexual men were less likely than heterosexual men (8.6% vs. 9.9%) to engage in heavy drinking in the past month.

Homelessness

- LGBTQ youth and young adults have a higher risk of experiencing homelessness.
  - This risk is especially high among Black LGBTQ youth.
  - Unstable housing is often the result of family rejection and discrimination based on their gender identity or sexual orientation.
  - Finding homeless shelters that will accept them can be difficult for this population and they experience elevated rates of harassment and abuse in these spaces.

Suicide

- The LGBTQ population is at an increased risk for suicidal thoughts and suicide attempts.
    - The rate of suicide attempts is four times greater for lesbian, gay, and bisexual youth and two times greater for questioning youth than that of heterosexual youth.
- High school students who identify as lesbian, gay, or bisexual are almost five times as likely to attempt suicide compared to their heterosexual peers.
- 40% of transgender adults have attempted suicide in their lifetime, compared to less than 5% of the general U.S. population.
    - Transgender individuals who identify as African American/black, Hispanic/Latino, American Indian/Alaska Native, or multiracial/mixed race are at increased risk of suicide attempts than white transgender individuals.

Fast Facts

LGBTQ people are at a higher risk for depression, anxiety, substance misuse, and suicide.

Access to Care

- The approach to sexual orientation and gender identity in mental health care can group together anyone in the LGBTQ community (even considered at all).
    - This method can be problematic as each subcommunity faces unique challenges, rates of mental illness, and experiences.
- The LGBTQ population is a wide range of individuals with separate and overlapping challenges regarding their behavioral health.
- The community also has other factors including race and economic status that can affect the quality of care they receive or their ability to access care.
- LGBTQ people face harassment or a lack of cultural competency from nurses and healthcare providers.
    - These experiences can lead those who receive treatment to fear disclosing their sexual orientation and/or gender identity due to potential discrimination or provider bias.

MENTAL HEALTH ASSESSMENT: CASE STUDIES

Case 1: Robyn: A Bisexual Woman

Robyn, a 28-year-old Black woman, presents to her primary care nurse practitioner (NP) with complaints of anxiety, hopelessness, and trouble sleeping. Robyn recently ended a relationship with a man, but she identifies as a bisexual woman. When she "came out" to her boyfriend, their relationship felt strained, and he did not fully understand her sexual orientation. Robyn feels comfortable with her bisexual orientation but wonders if there is something wrong with her. She has been in relationships with both men and women in the past. However, the people she dated—whether man or woman—were repeatedly less comfortable with Robyn's bisexuality. Robyn says that she feels "tired" of coming out to these people and fears that she will not find anyone who accepts her sexual orientation. Robyn's lesbian friends have also told her that it is time she makes up her mind whether she is a lesbian or straight and some have quit talking to her. She asks the NP for a sleep aid, as she cannot turn her mind off at night and the loneliness of her identity is getting to her.

- This scenario highlights the discrimination that bisexual people can face within the heterosexual and LGBTQ communities. Many bisexual people feel that they are not accepted by either the "straight" or LGBTQ communities. Some believe that bisexuality is a phase that one goes through.
- The NP should affirm with Robyn that being bisexual is not a mental health disorder and that the anxiety and hopelessness is an effect of the stigma and discrimination on being bisexual.
- As seen previously, the negative stereotypes and stigma about bisexuality impact the mental and physical health of Robyn. Research has shown that bisexual people have high rates of depression and anxiety when compared with gay and lesbian people (Mayer et al., 2015).
- The NP caring for Robyn should evaluate their own thoughts and beliefs about bisexual people and understand that while Robyn identifies with the LGBTQ community, that she has unique mental health needs that should be addressed.
  - To help Robyn, the NP should validate her experiences as real and refer Robyn to a mental health professional that specializes in bisexual people. It should not be assumed that all LGBTQ services are appropriate or available for bisexual people.

Bisexual patients are often not accepted by either the straight or LGBTQ communities and might present with their own unique behavioral health challenges.

CASE 2: BRENDA: DEPRESSION AND SUICIDE

Brenda is a 36-year-old transgender woman who presents to the ED for alcohol intoxication. She was found by medics and transported to the nearest facility. Brenda's vital signs are stable, but she is being admitted to the floor for further assessment about repeatedly telling the nursing staff to "leave me alone and just let me die."

The following day, Brenda is seen by the hospital's psychiatric nurse. The nurse questions Brenda about her life and alcohol use. Brenda reports that she has been depressed, backing out of events, not enjoying anything anymore, and spending most of her time drinking or seeking out alcohol. Several times throughout the interview, Brenda says everyone would be better off without her around and that she does not know how she can keep on living like this.

- *In this case, the RN should further inquire about Brenda's history with depression, has she been previously diagnosed, and whether this is her first episode and share this information with a psychiatrist to determine if Brenda is experiencing depression.*
  - *Depression can be difficult to diagnose in any patient. There are many causes for depression, and environmental stressors can be a trigger for LGBTQ people. The RN should not assume that Brenda is depressed because she is transgender but rather explore how her experiences of being transgender may have contributing factors to her current state.*
  - *Brenda's remarks about "everyone being better off without her" and that she does not know how she can keep living like this should be a trigger to RN as this could be a signal of suicidal ideation.*
  - *The RN should complete a thorough suicide assessment:*
    - *Ask directly if she has thought about hurting herself.*
      - *Ask directly if she has the means to harm themselves (such as access to weapons or a stockpile of pills).*

(continued)

(continued)

         o   *Are there events or goals that Brenda is looking forward to?*

         o   *A lack of looking forward to the future can be a warning sign for imminent risk of harm.*

       ❑ *Substance misuse can place someone like Brenda at a higher risk of impulsive behaviors that could result in harm.*

         o   *Past suicide attempts should be evaluated for lethality.*

       ❑ *If Brenda is found to have an active suicidal ideation with means and a plan, then an urgent psychiatric evaluation is warranted.*

- *When treating someone like Brenda, the RN not only should understand how sexual orientation or being transgender can affect symptoms but also should not assume that these factors manifest for all LGBTQ people. This can help the RN to create a therapeutic relationship with LGBTQ patients.*

- *Depressed LGBTQ people will respond better if they have a therapist, nurse, or healthcare provider who understands their concerns and works to create a safe space for them.*

The stress caused by stigma and discrimination can negatively impact their behavioral health of LGBTQ people. LGBTQ people with a behavioral health diagnosis have to manage both the stigma of being LGBTQ as well as the stigma of mental illnesses.

Fast Facts

- The stress caused by stigma and discrimination can negatively impact their behavioral health of LGBTQ people.

- LGBTQ people with a behavioral health diagnosis have to manage both the stigma of being LGBTQ as well as the stigma of mental illnesses.

- Bisexual patients are often not accepted by either the straight or LGBTQ communities and might present with their own unique behavioral health challenges.

- Nurses who work with LGBTQ people should provide them with care and communication that validates and affirms their identities.

- LGBTQ people are at a higher risk for depression, anxiety, substance misuse, and suicide.

Further Reading

Casanave, S. (2016, November 22). *Dealing with double stigma: The brink.* http://www.bu.edu/articles/2016/dealing-with-double-stigma

Mayer, K. H., Potter, J., Goldhammer, H., & Makadon, H. J. (2015). *The Fenway guide to lesbian, gay, bisexual, and transgender health.* American College of Physicians.

Miller, S. (2019, June 24). The young are regarded as the most tolerant generation. That's why results of this LGBTQ survey are 'alarming.' https://www.usatoday.com/story/news/nation/2019/06/24/lgbtq-acceptance-millennials-decline-glaad-survey/1503758001/

National Alliance on Mental Illness. (2020). *LGBTQI.* https://www.nami.org/Your-Journey/Identity-and-Cultural-Dimensions/LGBTQI

National Institute on Drug Abuse. (2020, August 25). *Substance use and suds in LGBTQ* populations.* https://www.drugabuse.gov/drug-topics/substance-use-suds-in-lgbtq-populations

Neighmond, P. (2020, May 17). *Home but not safe, some LGBTQ young people face rejection from families in lockdown.* https://www.npr.org/sections/health-shots/2020/05/17/856090474/home-but-not-safe-some-lgbtq-young-people-face-rejection-from-families-in-lockdo

Trevor Project. (2017, September 20). *Facts about suicide.* https://www.thetrevorproject.org/resources/preventing-suicide/facts-about-suicide/

Veltman, A., & Chaimowitz, G. (2014). Mental health care for people who identify as lesbian, gay, bisexual, transgender, and (or) queer. *Canadian Journal of Psychiatry. Revue canadienne de psychiatrie, 59*(11), 1–8.

Further Reading

III

LGBTQ Nursing Care and Implications

9

Self-Awareness and Bias

Humans naturally react with a wide range of emotions during strange encounters with people and situations. These reactions can range from positive and welcoming to negative and shocking. Nurses and providers might not even be aware of these reactions. To provide LGBTQ people with culturally competent care, we have to have an understanding of our own conscious and unconscious biases. This chapter will allow the nurse to understand their own internal biases in hopes better to raise self-awareness.

In this chapter, you will learn:

1. How biases can impact nurse–patient–provider relationships
2. The differences between conscious and unconscious bias
3. Ways to question and acknowledge biases and assumptions
4. Tips for self-discovery and growth

UNDERSTANDING BIAS

Bias can be defined as a tendency or inclination to prefer a person, idea, or thing over another. Biases are often based on stereotypes rather than an actual knowledge of a person or circumstances. Bias is divided into two subsets: conscious (explicit bias) or unconscious (implicit bias). Our biases about people are often from physical attributes such as ethnicity, gender, and age, as well as other attributes such as religion, sexual orientation, and gender identity.

Almost every impact of our lives shapes our biases. Our childhoods and family networks often serve as the foundation of biases. In today's age, a new force challenging and shaping our biases is social media.

Lifelong factors that impact biases are as follows:

- Religion
- Nationality
- Education
- Positive and negative life experiences
- Friends and family
- Coworkers
- Employment

Throughout our days, we encounter and process thousands, if not millions, of pieces of information, and our brain simply cannot process all of that information at once. Instead, our minds make snap judgments based on our biases. These reactions guide us through situations that are both familiar and unfamiliar and will dictate how we treat others—whether positively or negatively.

Bias in Nursing

We start to put the patient into categories and boxes the minute we see each other. This bias can begin even before we meet the person, only by their intake information. During our interactions with patients, we shape and allow our bias to take charge in deciding whether we can relate to this patient or if we perceive them as an "other."

Patient factors affecting bias in nursing are as follows:

- Age
- Body size
- Gender
- Skin color
- The appearance of their clothing
- Mannerism
- Medical history

The challenge during these situations is to stop categorizing, controlling, and predicting our patients' identities so we are open in our communication. As nurses, we want to go into clinical situations open to every possibility with every patient. Identifying our assumptions and biases requires constant and deliberate vigilance as those assumptions often arise from unconscious bias.

LGBTQ Bias

Bias toward LGBTQ people continues to change, as does society's perception and embracement of LGBTQ people. Bias can be overt, such as derogatory terms and prejudice, or subtle, such as through microaggressions, disinterest, and disengagement. Although in the United States we have seen changes in mainstream media, the repeal of "Don't Ask, Don't Tell," and the Supreme Court decision that legalized same sex marriage in 2016, LGBTQ people still face high rates of violence and discrimination in healthcare and their daily lives.

Bias toward LGBTQ people can harm the nurse–patient relationship and perpetuate the health disparities this population faces. This bias can play out in our communication, body language, and assessments of our patients. Unconsciously or consciously, biased nurses miss essential details about a person's health history and impact our interactions and clinical decision-making.

Nurses, like most people, may resist the idea that they are biased toward LGBTQ people. Some may say that they have friends or family who are LGBTQ, that they are a member of the LGBTQ community, or even something like, "I don't see what the big deal is, LGBTQ people have it much easier nowadays."

However, a 2015 study based on data from the Sexuality Implicit Assessment Test (IAT) found that heterosexual sexual physicians, nurses, and other healthcare providers implicitly favored heterosexual people over gay and lesbian people. Additionally, another study found that 38% of gay and lesbian people had preferences for heterosexual. These preferences or biases shape not only our interactions with our patients and peers but also how we create our healthcare systems, design forms, and our nursing education and practice.

For transgender patients, our bias can lead us to reject or distance ourselves from patients. Many nurses cannot relate to being born in the wrong body; thus, they are unable to connect to a transgender person. Nurses may view transgender people as entirely foreign, damaging the therapeutic relationship and creating barriers to effective communication.

CONSCIOUS VERSUS UNCONSCIOUS BIAS

Freud uses the metaphor of an iceberg to describe our conscious and unconscious mind. The tip of the iceberg that is floating above the water is our conscious bias. These are thoughts, feelings, and memories that readily come to mind. Our unconscious mind is the bottom of the iceberg below the sea—unseen and inaccessible to the consciousness. Still, it profoundly influences judgments, feelings, and behaviors.

Conscious (or explicit) bias is considered to be aware, intentional, and responsive. If people perceive their conscious biases to be valid, they are more likely to engage in unfair treatment or violence. Research has shown conscious bias reduced when people have experiences and contact with people outside their group. Expressions of conscious bias happen as a result of deliberate thought processes. As nurses, we must be aware of these conscious biases so that we can regulate them actively and disrupt negative or prejudicial thoughts.

Unconscious biases (or implicit bias) are learned stereotypes that are automatic, unintentional, and they can affect our behaviors. Unconscious bias, if left unchecked, can be dangerous. This type of bias impacts decisions on recruitment and hiring, access to healthcare, and can even impact outcomes in criminal justice cases. Remember unconscious biases are not permanent and are malleable.

Fast Facts

Unconscious (or implicit) biases are unquestioned or instinctive assumptions about an individual based on their association with a particular group.

Unconscious Bias and LGBTQ

Unconscious bias toward LGBTQ people can lead the nurse to associate certain risk factors, such as unsafe sexual behaviors, with LGBTQ subgroups such as gay men but not with others such as lesbians. These assumptions can result in rapid, unfounded judgments that can ultimately affect our interaction or communication with our patients (e.g., assume a gay man has multiple partners when he is actually in a monogamous relationship).

If a nurse is unwilling to engage in self-inquiry of their own biases or encounter a provider who is unable to change their perspectives toward interactions with LGBTQ patients, we must remember our ethical and moral obligation to do no harm. It is critical in these situations that nurses and other providers be honest with themselves and the patient and make a referral to a nurse or clinician who will be able to treat the patient with respect and compassion.

Fast Facts

Unconscious biases are automatic and can affect our behaviors and interactions. These biases can be changed through active reflection and discussion.

UNDERSTANDING AND ACKNOWLEDGING BIASES

To understand your own bias and assumptions and societal stigma toward LGBTQ people, Exhibit 9.1 can be used as a self-assessment for insight. This test was created by Peggy Macintosh to explore the effects of white privilege. Still, it can be tailored to explore the bias of many minority groups.

Exhibit 9.1

Self-Assessment Test to Demonstrate the Effect of External Bias (Heterosexual Privilege)

Daily, as a straight person:

- I can go for months without being called straight.
- I am not asked to think about why I am straight.
- I am never asked to speak for everyone who is heterosexual.
- People do not ask why I chose to be heterosexual.
- People do not ask why I made my choice to be public about my sexual orientation.
- Nobody calls me straight as an insult.
- When I talk about heterosexuality (such as a joke or talking about my relationships), I will not be accused of pushing my sexual orientation onto others.
- I do not have to fear that if my family or friends find out about my heterosexuality, there will be economic, emotional, physical, or psychological consequences.
- I can be sure my classes will require curricular materials that testify to the existence of people with my sexual orientation.
- I can easily find a religious community that will not exclude me for being heterosexual.
- I can count on finding a therapist or doctor willing and able to talk about my sexuality.
- I am guaranteed to find sex education literature for couples with my sexual orientation.
- Because of my sexual orientation, I do not need to worry that people will harass or assault me.
- I am not identified/defined by my sexual orientation.
- I can hold hands or kiss my significant other in public and not have people double-take or stare.
- I can be open about my sexual orientation without worrying about my job.

Source: Adapted from https://njdc.info/wp-content/uploads/2013/11/invisible _knapsack2a.pdf

TIPS FOR NAVIGATING BIAS

Navigating biases and assumptions cannot be done overnight. It is a journey we are consistently undertaking. Be willing to step outside of your comfort zones for growth. Look inward and understand your worldview and beliefs. This type of introspection can be difficult. For some, it can lead to feelings of guilt, shame, and questioning of their belief system but can take comfort knowing that they are not alone in this journey and their clinical practice and relationships can become enriched because of this process.

1. Self-Awareness
   a. The first step to address bias is to promote self-awareness. What are our biases, and where do they stem from? There are many instruments available on the internet to assess one's bias. Nurses who are curious about their own biases and want to become more self-aware, the IAT is available online and can be taken for free at https://implicit.harvard.edu.
2. Be Mindful of Language
   a. Our words help to shape our thoughts and perceptions of this world. Take the word, queer—once a derogatory term, it is now used as an identity for many people around the world.
   b. How we ask questions and respond can set a precedent for the entire interaction with the patient. Are we making assumptions about the patient (e.g., if they are a female, is it assumed they have a husband if they are married?)
   c. Does your tone (voice and body) convey positive or negative?
3. Encourage peers to call our bias and hold each other accountable (see Box 9.1)
   a. Serve as a role model.
   b. Seek out clarifying information when insensitive comments are made about LGBTQ patients—is this intentional or unintentional? Some people may have a lack of understanding, whereas others can be overtly hurtful. Either situation can lead to patients not being treated with dignity and respect and harming the nurse–patient relationship for future encounters.
   c. Always remember that the goal is never to start an argument or hostility. People may have their own beliefs, but anti-LGBTQ remarks and jokes cannot be tolerated in healthcare environments. Nurses must advocate for and create an atmosphere of dignity and respect.
4. Seek training and educational experiences

a. Look for educational opportunities to learn more about LGBTQ people and other diverse populations that may be prone to bias.

b. Unconscious bias training can help people better understand biases and their selves.

CASE STUDY 1

Anthony is meeting his pregnant wife, Mpande, for a prenatal appointment with the midwife. Anthony is transgender and is in the process of transitioning from female to male.

The midwife, along with a midwife student, enters the room and sees Anthony. She says to Anthony, "Hi, you must be Mpande's sister. It's nice to meet you!"

Anthony, upset, responds, "No, I am her husband."

The midwife looks startled and mumbles, "Oh, sorry."

The student notices that Anthony and Mpande are visibly uncomfortable, but he does not say anything.

1. *Why are Anthony and Mpande upset in this scenario?*
   a. *This interaction included a bias based on heteronormativity, as the midwife assumed that Anthony was Mpande's sister, as opposed to her spouse. These implicit biases made Anthony feel "invisible" and unwelcome. It is important not to make any assumptions about the relationship between the patients and the people they bring with them.*
   b. *The midwife assumed that Anthony was Mpande's sister based on Anthony's gender presentation. This mistaken assumption was hurtful because Anthony identifies as male.*
2. *How could the midwife have responded instead?*
   a. *"Hi, it is nice to meet you. What are your names, and what is your relationship to each other?"*
3. *How could the student have talked to the midwife preceptor about the interaction?*
   a. *Discussions about biased behavior can be stressful for anyone. The midwife may respond defensively, which can be challenging. It is important to evaluate the risk of responding in these situations. If the student feels safe, they can follow-up with their preceptor directly in a private space and let them know that what they observed, how the assumption could have been avoided, and how she might have apologized more emphatically.*
   b. *The student could open the discussion, with a statement such as, "I'm sure you didn't mean to be hurtful, but when you..."*

BOX 9.1 TIPS FOR NAVIGATING DISCUSSIONS ABOUT BIASED BEHAVIORS

- Using "I" statements instead of "you" statements
- Separating intent from impact
- Appealing to empathy
- Focusing on kindness, respect, and obligation

CASE STUDY 2

Becca is a nursing student who has to receive a physical examination for her nursing program. Becca identifies as pansexual and, during the examination, the family nurse practitioner made comments about her sexuality, saying, "Is that what all the young kids are calling it these days? It's impossible to keep up with all this stuff. Maybe I'm just old, but it seems like everyone is just confused. I don't remember dealing with all this when I was younger."

1. *How did the nurse practitioner's interaction highlight a lack of self-awareness and potential bias?*
   a. *The nurse practitioner might be trying to be casual and approachable with Becca; however, in this scenario, they may be sending a message that Becca's sexuality is not to be taken seriously.*
   b. *Becca could interpret their words as a rejection of her identity. This can greatly diminish patient–provider trust and can make her less likely to be open with future providers.*
2. *What could the nurse practitioner have said instead?*
   a. *Having self-awareness about their own biases in regard to sexuality and the various identities that a person may have will enable the provider to create a therapeutic and trusting relationship. When encountering clinical situation such as this, nurses and other providers should pause before commenting about something that they are unfamiliar with.*
   b. *Rather than being dismissive about Becca's sexual identity, they can ask Becca to explain in her own words what being pansexual means to her. The provider may also want to educate themselves through continuing education and reliable resources about different terms that people use to identify their sexuality. After an encounter such as this, it is important for providers to reflect on the encounter and how their self-awareness and biases played a role and how they can work to improve future encounters.*

Source: Adapted and revised from the LGBTQIA Health Education Center. https://www.lgbtqiahealtheducation.org

Fast Facts

Biases toward LGBTQ people can be overt (discrimination and prejudice) or it can be subtle (communication, body language, clinical decisions) through our interactions as healthcare providers.

Further Reading

Carabez, R., Pellegrini, M., Mankovitz, A., Eliason, M., Ciano, M., & Scott, M. (2015). "Never in all my years...": Nurses' education about LGBT health. *Journal of Professional Nursing, 31*(4), 323–329. https://doi.org/10.1016/j.profnurs.2015.01.003

Foglia, M., & Goldsen, K. (2014). Health disparities among LGBT older adults and the role of nonconscious bias. *Hastings Centers Report, 44*(5), 40–44. https://doi.org/10.1002/hast.369

McDowell, M. J., Goldhammer, H., Potter, J. E., & Keuroghlian, A. S. (2020). Strategies to mitigate clinician implicit bias against sexual and gender minority patients. *Psychosomatics, 61*(6), 655–661. https://doi.org/10.1016/j.psym.2020.04.021

Myaer, K. H., Potter, J., Goldhammer, H., & Makadon, H. J. (2015). *The Fenway guide to lesbian, gay, bisexual, and transgender health.* American College of Physicians.

Sabin, J., Riskind, R., & Nosek, B. (2015). Health care providers' implicit and explicit attitudes toward lesbian women and gay men. *American Journal of Public Health, 105*(9), 1831–1841. https://doi.org/10.2105/AJPH.2015.302631

Singer, R. (2015). LGBTQ focused education: Can inclusion be taught? *International Journal of Childbirth Education, 30*(2), 17–19.

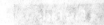

10

Communication Best Practices

Communication is key to providing culturally competent nursing care to LGBTQ people. Understanding basic terminologies and communicating will help to build a therapeutic relationship with the patient. This chapter is a toolbox of communication techniques to help guide the nurse to communicate with compassion.

In this chapter, you will learn:

1. The importance of communicating with affirmation and support
2. How to create compassionate relationships with LGBTQ people
3. Techniques and insights to create a communication "toolbox"

COMMUNICATING WITH AFFIRMATION AND SUPPORT

It is not always apparent to the nurse or provider if their patient identifies as LGBTQ. Making assumptions about the identities of our patients can negatively impact the relationship with the patient. High-quality patient–clinician communication has been shown to improve patient engagement, satisfaction, and overall adherence to care plans. Using the right words can build trust and help to gain the confidence of the patient. Using the wrong words or avoiding effective communication with LGBTQ people can cause unnecessary barriers and shut down lines of communication, which can have far-lasting implications, even outside of healthcare.

Communication is critical to the health and well-being of LGBTQ people. Communicating in a nonjudgmental and in an open style will allow patients to express themselves freely.

THE BASICS FOR A COMMUNICATION "TOOLBOX"

- Accept each patient as their unique individual and identity.
  - Do not make assumptions about gender identity, sexuality, and relationship status.
  - Assure confidentiality.
- Use terms that the person calls themselves.
  - If they use the term "gay," do not refer to them as "homosexual" during the encounter.
  - This can feel awkward at first—that is okay!
- Maintain a nonjudgmental attitude.
  - Avoid showing surprise or disapproval.
  - Check facial expressions and body language.
- Avoid using words that assume the person has a partner or parents that are the opposite sex. This is important because the patient may fear that you will judge them if they do not respond appropriately.
  - Instead of asking "What are the names of your mother and father?" ask "What are the names of your parents?"
  - Instead of "Do you have a husband or boyfriend?" try "Are you in a relationship?"
- Use the correct gender pronouns and chosen name when referring to a patient.
  - It is not possible to guess a person's gender identity based off of their name or by how they look or sound.
  - Ask for their gender pronouns on intake and during the assessment.
    - "I would like to be respectful. How would you like to be addressed?"
    - "What names/pronouns would you like me/us to use?"
    - If appropriate, incorporate your own pronouns into your introduction and/or include them on your badge.
  - When addressing a patient for the first time, avoid using pronouns that invoke a gender—simply say, "How may I help you?" Instead of "How may I help you, sir?"

- It is acceptable to use "they" instead of "he" or "she" in the singular form.
  - Instead of "He is here for his 3 o'clock appointment," try "They are here for their 3 o'clock appointment."
  - *Never* refer to a person as an "it."

Fast Facts

It is nearly impossible to assume someone's gender or sexual identity from appearance or sound.

- Avoid unnecessary questions.
  - Ask yourself, "Is this question necessary for the patient's care, or am I asking this question for my curiosity?"
- Be kind to yourself.
  - It is okay to make mistakes. Apologize and learn.
- It is okay not to be an expert.
  - Be honest and open.
  - Find the information if you are unsure.
  - No one is ever truly an expert, as culture and society are fluid and ever changing.
- Do not go at this alone.
  - Share discomforts with others and celebrate successes.
- Remember that your behaviors and interactions set the examples for others. Interact and lead with integrity.

CASE STUDY: JOHN

At a primary care office, the nurse is helping John, a teenage boy, with his check-in for a new visit. While entering the intake form into the health record, the nurse notices that John left the parent section blank. The nurse says to John, "What are the names of your mother and father? You didn't complete that section."

> *John averts his eyes and says softly, "I have two dads. Their names are Luke and Dennis."*
>
> *Without hesitating, the nurse says, "Oh! Don't you have a mother?" John quickly flushes, and he appears very uncomfortable.*

(continued)

(continued)

Discussion: In this scenario, the nurse assumed John has opposite-sex parents. This is probably something that John faces routinely, and he has most likely been treated differently because of this. He is not ashamed of his parents but tries to avoid awkward situations with people who do not understand his family dynamic. Using the communication techniques listed earlier, the nurse could have created an open and welcoming environment for John and invited him to talk more about his parents by removing the gender implications of asking about his mother and father. Although this is seemingly innocent, these assumptions and biases can impact the patient's relationship with the nurse.

CASE STUDY

Carl Jones, a transgender man, is being admitted to the hospital for a routine chemotherapy admission and is joined by his wife. Since Carl is still in the process of legally changing his name, all of his records are still under his previous name of Carla.

The nurse comes to Carl's room to complete the admission assessment. The nurse approaches Carl's wife and begins the assessment, asking Carla to confirm her name and birthday.

Carl's wife states that she is not the patient and that Carl is sitting over there.

The nurse apologizes for the mistake and turns to Carl. The nurse confirms the name of Carla Jones with Carl then tells him that she will make a note entry into the system with his chosen name. The nurse further explains to Carl that, although his name is recorded, there may be times where the staff will have to use Carla for safety purposes, as that is what matches his legal documents.

Carl tells the nurse that he appreciates the information and the nurse for taking the time to explain to him about his name.

Discussion: In this situation, the nurse promptly acknowledged their mistake of identifying the patient. The nurse further engaged the patient by asking about their chosen name and committing to make sure the healthcare team and medical record were updated with that knowledge. By educating Carl about safety measures in place in the hospital and why healthcare staff may occasionally use the former name, the nurse validated Carl while also being transparent about expectations. While staff should be respectful and use Carl's chosen name during interactions, there may be times, where his former name has to be used for safety purposes—that is, medication administration, patient identification.

Fast Facts

Effective communication is a crucial step to eliminating LGBTQ health disparities.

Communicating with LGBTQ people requires not only understanding the population as a whole but also understanding the individuality and uniqueness of each person. By using these communication techniques, the nurse will be better prepared to communicate effectively not only with LGBTQ patients but with all people they encounter. By taking these steps, the nurse will ensure that all people are treated with the dignity and respect that they deserve.

Further Reading

Levitt, N., & Reiss, E. (n.d.). *Enhancing your clinical skills in caring for LGBTQ patients.* Retrieved January 17, 2021, from https://www.hss.edu/conditions_enhancing-clinical-skills-LGBTQ-care-hospital-setting.asp

Mayer, K. H., Potter, J., Goldhammer, H., & Makadon, H. J. (2015). *The Fenway guide to lesbian, gay, bisexual, and transgender health.* American College of Physicians.CH10 Communication Best Practices

11

History and Physical Examination of LGBTQ

Taking an LGBTQ inclusive health history and culturally competent physical examination is the foundation of nursing and medical care. The goal of this chapter is to help guide nurses to improve the quality of their interactions with LGBTQ patients. The history and physical examination that nurses complete is one of the most pivotal moments in the nurse–patient relationship. Many nurses make assumptions about sexuality and gender identity, and most guides have been designed without LGBTQ people in mind. This chapter explores how the nurse can conduct a culturally competent health assessment and physical examination.

In this chapter, you will learn:

1. How to improve the quality of interactions with LGBTQ people
2. How to build and establish a trusting relationship with LGBTQ patients
3. How to conduct a physical assessment with dignity and respect

Nurses and healthcare providers use various methods to collect and interpret data about their patients. This can be in the form of intake and registration forms, electronic charting, interview templates, physical assessments, laboratory values, and many others. This data collection allows the nurse to understand the health needs of their patient and how they can best deliver care in that setting. Unfortunately, many forms and templates in place do not acknowledge LGBTQ people and their needs. They often lead the nurse to assumptions and biases. This chapter will provide some basics for the nurse to better understand the nuances of LGBTQ care and how they can tailor their history and physical examination to be culturally competent and sensitive.

Note, while this chapter highlights some of the differences of LGBTQ people, there are many ways in which LGBTQ people are similar to all other patients. Many LGBTQ people experience life and share the same health concerns as the rest of the general population. The information provided here is to help the nurse to build a compassionate and trusting relationship with LGBTQ patients.

INTAKE AND REGISTRATION FORMS

Often, the first impression that a patient can have of the healthcare experience. For LGBTQ people, this can set the tone of whether their personal information and identities are important and worthwhile to the practice/hospital/etc.

- Replace terms such as "marital status" with "relationship status" and/or acknowledge that same-sex relationships are legitimate and valued.
- Use the term "partner" and other gender-neutral or inclusive language whenever possible.
- Use open-ended responses to questions whenever possible.
  - For gender, leave a space for people to self-identify if they feel that the given options do not apply.
- Include sexual orientation and gender identity on every form registration or intake form.
  - Normalizes the collection of this data.
  - Shows LGBTQ people that this data is essential to the nurse and providers.
  - Allows healthcare organizations to collect data to serve diverse populations better.
  - People are more likely to disclose their identities on a form, rather than a spontaneous question by a nurse.
- Share confidentiality statement with every patient with their intake and registration.

FACE-TO-FACE INTERVIEW

Approach the face-to-face interview with open-mindedness and without judgment. It is essential to elicit information about the patient's sexual orientation, gender identity, and sexual practices. Depending on the situation and context, it could also be prudent to inquire about their previous experiences with healthcare providers. This will allow the nurse to understand better their experiences and how they can help to rebuild trust in the healthcare system.

- Do not make assumptions about literacy, language, and comfort with direct communication.
- Do not assume that being LGBTQ is always hard. Many LGBTQ people are well adjusted and live their lives with the same stresses as the heterosexual and cisgender populations.
- Remember that it is impossible to avoid assumptions, and mistakes will inevitably be made. Always apologize right away and acknowledge the error.
- Listen to the patient and how they describe their gender and sexuality.
  - Reflect and use their choice of language.
  - Some people may call themselves queer, but for other LGBTQ patients, they may have encountered this word used in a derogatory manner.
- Be mindful of body language and facial expressions.
- Ask open-ended questions.

HEALTH HISTORY

Personal and family health history and screenings can provide valuable information for the nurse to understand the person's past and current health. All patients, regardless if LGBTQ or not, should have the followed assessed:

- History of present illness
- Review of systems
- Medical history
- Medications and allergies
- Family history

As mentioned in previous chapters, LGBTQ people are at a higher risk for specific medical, behavioral health problems when compared to the general population. It is believed that most of these health disparities are the result and consequence of high levels of exposure to societal stigma and discrimination.

LGBTQ health history must include questions about sexual orientation and gender identity. This information is important to show awareness and acceptance and avoid misdiagnosis and improper care and treatment.

Considerations for the LGBTQ Health History

- A detailed vaccination history should be obtained from all LGBTQ patients, and vaccines should be updated as per recommendations from the Advisory Committee on Immunization Practice.
  - Essential vaccines for the LGBTQ people include:
    - HPV vaccine for all youth up to age 26
- Hepatitis A and B vaccine for those who engage in high-risk sexual activities or injection drug use.
- Body image
  - Body image and weight can affect members of the LGBTQ differently
    - Some gay/bisexual men struggle with body image and may be more likely to experience eating disorders, engage in excessive exercise, or use substances to achieve a more masculine/muscular appearance than their heterosexual counterparts.
    - Many lesbians reject traditional cultural norms surrounding beauty and thinness. Lesbians are more likely to be overweight; thus, it is important to approach the topic with compassion and care.
    - This is an ideal opportunity for providers to understand their transgender patient's views of their bodies and begin the discussion about medical transition.
- Spirituality
  - Many LGBTQ people find significant strength or hope from spiritual practice. Even though some traditional organizations have rejected LGBTQ people, many welcome LGBTQ people, which allows the nurse to provide them with appropriate resources for this journey.
- Family and relationships
  - Relationships can serve as a source of social support, a stressor, or both.
  - LGBTQ people face high risks of being alienated from biological families.

- This rejection can take a toll on mental health.
- LGBTQ youth are at a higher risk of suicide and mental health concerns from the risk of the rejection of friends and family.
  - LGBTQ youth represent roughly 40% of the homeless youth population. Studies have shown that upward of 60% of homeless LGBTQ youth are likely to attempt suicide.
- Important to know that LGBTQ may have "families of choice."
  - Networks of support that function as a family but without the relation of blood or marriage
- Advance directives
  - LGBTQ people are more likely to choose a friend or nonlegally recognized partner.
  - Ensure the person has the document officially completed so it will be upheld under the law if and when the advanced directive is needed.
- Mental health
  - LGBTQ people face higher rates of depression, anxiety, and self-harm behaviors.
  - Establish trust with the LGBTQ patient to assess their mental health because they may be "hiding" parts of themselves and/or disconnected to social support systems.
  - Be familiar with local LGBTQ-friendly mental health providers in your area.
- Substance use
  - LGBTQ people are more likely to use alcohol and drugs, have higher rates of substance abuse, and continue heavy drinking later into life.
  - Assess LGBTQ people in a thorough and thoughtful manner.
    - This assessment could arouse feelings of shame or denial in the patient.
  - Be willing to address openly and encourage support.
  - Behavioral change is a process that may require regular check-ins over many visits or years.
    - Schedule frequent touchpoints to encourage continued smoking cessation, decreased alcohol consumption, and other substance use.
- Safety and social issues
  - For LGBTQ people, safety and social issues can be extremely complex depending on the patient's acceptance of their own identity and their experience with minority stress.
    - An individual's connectedness and level of identification may correlate with health outcomes—higher levels of

"outness" has been shown to decrease risky sexual behaviors and improve mental health.

- ❑ Consider implementing questions to probe for the effects of social stress on their health.
- Sexual history
  - Taking a thorough sexual history communicates to the patient that sexual health is an integral part of their health and opens up communication about sexual concerns or questions they may have.
  - Body language, the framing and reception of the questions, and the introduction of the questions will influence the assessment.
  - Begin with a statement that these questions are asked of all patients and vital to their overall health.
  - Avoid the presumption of heterosexuality.
  - Do not assume that because a person identifies as gay or lesbian that they do not have sexual encounters (whether past, present, or future) with the opposite sex.
  - Incorporate sex education and risk mitigation into the discussion.

Fast Facts

LGBTQ-specific concerns to be addressed during the health assessment include mental health, preventative screenings, body image, sexual health, and social support.

- Transgender-specific considerations
  - What names and pronouns do you prefer?
  - What sex were you assigned at birth?
  - How would you describe your gender identity?
  - Inquire about any changes in their appearance or body.
  - Ask about the use of medications or hormones to change their gender presentation.
  - Assess for physical, sexual, or emotional violence.
  - Gauge their readiness or desire for surgeries.

PHYSICAL EXAMINATION

All nurses are trained on how to complete a physical examination; however, it is important to understand how the examination may be done sensitively for LGBTQ patients. A physical examination of parts of the body, such as the breasts, genitals, and anus, can be intimidating and especially challenging to those individuals who experience body shame. This shame could be the result of body image issues, such as people with obesity, or from people who are experiencing gender dysphoria due to the existence of organs that do not align with their gender identity.

Considerations and recommendations for a comprehensive physical examination:

- Educate the patient on the why of the physical examination. Why do you as a provider have to complete this physical examination? Let them know that it helps us to better understand their bodies, assess for abnormalities, and ensure well-being.
- Ask the patient what language they would prefer for you to use to refer to their anatomy—that is, chest, breasts, pectorals.
- Ask the patient what might make them feel more comfortable:
  - Have a different provider perform the examination (i.e., a different gender).
  - Ask if they would like to include a support person.
  - Avoid language that has sexual or violent connotations (you will feel a prick, or "blades" or "stirrups").
  - Offering draping alternatives.
- Assure the patient they will be able to stop the examination at any time.
- Always obtain permission to proceed with the examination.
- Clarify the role of everyone in the room.
  - If the medical assistant is present, say why are they necessary and give the patient the option of choosing the gender of the individual.
- Warn the patient before performing all examination maneuvers, "I will now place the stethoscope on your chest to listen to your breath and heart."
- Speak in a calm and reassuring voice.

Transgender Considerations for the Physical Examination

For a successful physical examination, establishing a partnership with the patient is key. While completion of a routine physical examination is quickly second nature to the nurse, it can leave the patient with feelings of worry or unease. This is especially true for patients on the transgender spectrum (see Table 11.1). These patients should not only receive screenings and treatment based on their current anatomy but also understand the importance of their natal anatomy in their health assessment. The nurse should

Table 11.1

Transgender Patient Key Physical Examination Notes		
Transgender female	Tucking	Concern for urinary reflux/infections (epididymo-orchitis, prostatitis, cystitis)
	Genitourinary examination	• Use an anoscope for patients who have undergone surgery with vaginoplasty • Take extra care to explain each step, especially for patients who have not undergone surgery
	Prostate examination	Do not forget your patient may need a prostate exam
Transgender male	Binding	Concern for rib fractures, atelectasis, pneumonia
	Genitourinary examination	Use smallest speculum possible, with adequate lubrication
	Pregnancy test	Do not forget your patient may need a pregnancy test

Source: EMRA Transgender Care Guide. Reprinted by permission from Emergency Medicine Residents' Association.

recognize that some physical examinations may be difficult for those whose gender identity does not match anatomical parts. A culturally competent nurse can use the previous tips to ensure they assess their patients with dignity and respect.

Fast Facts

Transgender individuals have unique nuances and considerations to their physical assessment that the nurse should consider to be sensitive and safe.

The health history and physical examination are the foundations on which the nurses base their care off for the patient. For LGBTQ people, there are unique considerations that the nurse needs to know so that they can provide culturally competent care to LGBTQ people. Using the information in this chapter can help guide the nurse in these situations. Partnering with LGBTQ people in their health history and physical assessments develops a level of trust in which the patient may feel safe and respected—some for the first time.

CASE STUDY: AN INTERSEX PATIENT

Toby is 36-year-old patient who presents to the family health center to establish care. On the intake form, Toby checks the following:

a. *Sexual orientation: Choose not to disclose*
b. *Gender identity: Other—nonbinary*
c. *Sex assigned at birth: Female, other*

Toby's medical questionnaire mentions pediatric surgeries, unsure of last gynecological examinations, and mentions previous hormonal therapy.

What other information would the nurse caring for Toby want to know?

- *The nurse should begin the interview by asking Toby about pronouns. This is important for all patients, but Toby self-identified as nonbinary knowing Toby's pronouns would be an important step in establishing a trusting and therapeutic patient–nurse relationship.*
- *The nurse and provider should further explore Toby's disclosure of their sex assigned at birth.*

The nurse asks Toby about pronouns, and Toby tells the nurse that they go by they/them/theirs. The nurse then asks about their sex assigned at birth, and Toby discloses that they were born as intersex but underwent procedures as an infant to be a female. Toby mentions that she had previously taken estrogen as a child and adolescent but was not sure if she should continue taking it so she stopped in her 20s.

What other questions should the nurse and provider explore at this time?

- *Current health—ask questions about their own goals for health and well-being*
- *Family history*
- *Wellness and body image*
  - *Exercise and diet*
  - *How do they feel in their body?*
  - *Is there anything that they would want to change?*
- *Family and relationships*
  - *Who do you consider to be your family?*
  - *What does your social circle look like?*
- *Behavioral health*
- *Substance use*
  - *Ask about substances, type, how often, and situation that they would consume substances—that is, are you alone or with other people?*

(continued)

(continued)

- *Safety and social stressors*
  - *Knowing that Toby is intersex and nonbinary, it would be important to probe for minority stress*
    - *Are you comfortable with your friends, family, coworkers knowing about your gender identity?*
    - *Has anyone ever threatened you?*
    - *Do you conceal your identity?*
- *Sexual history*
  - *Avoid that language that presumes heterosexuality*
  - *Do not make assumptions*
  - *Assess for type of sexual activity, protection, and concerns*
  - *Assure confidentiality*

The RN completes the health history with Toby. The RN talks to Toby about the next steps of the visit, including the physician's assessment, verification of information, and the physical examination. During this discussion, the RN notices that Toby appears uncomfortable and asks if there is anything wrong at the moment. Toby mentions that sometimes they feel like an exhibit when people find out that they were born intersex and complete unnecessary physical examinations. They ask if the physical examination is necessary and if the physician could just see them and leave.

What steps should the RN take next to provide Toby with culturally competent care and ease Toby's concerns?

- *The nurse should ask and validate Toby's experiences with the examination.*
- *Use this time to educate Toby about the reasons that it is important for the examination to be completed and what the examination would entail if they decide to proceed. Furthermore, as this is their first encounter and if it is deemed not necessary, allow Toby to defer any intrusive assessment until another time or with a specialist, such as a gynecologist.*
- *Ask Toby if there is anything about their body that they should know or if there is any language that they wish for the nurse and doctor to use during the examination.*
- *Ask Toby what would make the examination more comfortable.*
- *Provide Toby with the assurance that they will be able to stop the examination at any time.*

Toby mentions that they feel that they developed a good relationship with the RN through their discussion and if they would be able to stay during the interactions with the physician. The nurse recognizes that this is a moment where Toby is establishing trust with the nurse and that it is important to support Toby during this time to ensure that their health needs are met. The nurse offers to stay with the examination and tells Toby that they will speak with the physician prior to the examination. The physician completes the physical examination with the RN and Toby leaves expressing satisfaction with the visit and schedules a follow-up appointment.

This case example highlights the importance of partnering with patients. This creates a trust that can transform a dreaded examination and interaction into an experience of safety and respect. Nurses, at any level, who build trusting relationships with their patients have the opportunity to provide an experience that is corrective and healing. With this trust and positive experiences, nurses can help to improve the health and well-being of LGBTQ people by conducting an LGBTQ-inclusive health history and culturally competent physical examination.

Further Reading

Mayer, K. H., Potter, J., Goldhammer, H., & Makadon, H. J. (2015). *The Fenway guide to lesbian, gay, bisexual, and transgender health.* American College of Physicians.

Trevor Project. (2018, July 9). *Youth homelessness.* https://www.thetrevor project.org/get-involved/trevor-advocacy/homelessness/

12

Transgender Health and Nursing Care

When discussing LGBTQ people, it is often assumed that people understand the differences between subpopulations. This "lumping" or broad use of LGBTQ can lead to inaccurate or incorrect beliefs about transgender people and further complicate their health and well-being. This chapter aims to highlight the distinctions of transgender people, acknowledge the diversity among trans people, define terms, and provide the reader with a deeper understanding of transgender health and nursing care.

In this chapter, you will learn:

1. About the unique health needs of the transgender population
2. A deeper understanding of transgender people
3. Barriers that transgender people face in accessing healthcare
4. Nursing considerations to deliver culturally competent care to transgender people.

TRANSGENDER—A DEEPER DIVE

In the United States, it is difficult to estimate the size of the transgender population accurately. There is no consistent data collection method to capture this population due to the diversity of population, legal and social implications, and the hidden nature of the transgender community. The U.S. census does not ask questions related to gender identity, and no significant national sampling or survey on this population has been completed. Legal protections for transgender people vary by country and even change state by state in the United States. This lack of protection makes data collection on sensitive populations difficult and almost impossible—people may fear the loss of housing, job, and/or family, or social support if their information is shared with various parties. Estimates about the transgender population can be made through the collection of data through *Diagnostic and Statistical Manual of Mental Disorders (DSM)* codes, data on suicide, tobacco use, and HIV rates among the trans community as well as from data of some ED visits or state health departments.

Current estimates on the size of the transgender population range from 0.1% to 0.5% of the population. It is believed the transgender population is "on the rise" as people, especially trans youth, feel supported to identify as transgender. This increase is important to nursing and healthcare because it is further proof that transgender people are not "rare" but rather a natural subset of the human population.

Gender Dysphoria

- A conflict between a person's assigned gender at birth and the gender in which they identify.
- People will sometimes describe that they are uncomfortable with their body or with the expected roles of their assigned gender.
- They may feel clinically significant distress or impairment due to a noncongruence of their gender role and gender identity.

Gender Transition/Gender Affirmation

The process of coming to recognize, accept, and express one's gender identity.

- Most often refers to the period when a person makes changes that others can see (e.g., changes to appearance, changes to their name and gender presentation).
- Called *gender affirmation* because it allows people to affirm their gender identity by making outward changes.
- Involves social, medical, legal components.
- Gender affirmation can significantly improve a person's mental and general well-being.
- *There is no one way to affirm one's gender.*

Table 12.1

Trans Definitions	
Transgender/trans	Individuals who have a gender identity not entirely congruent with their assigned sex at birth
Gender minority	A person who identifies as transgender, gender nonconforming, and/or whose gender identity or expressions differ from the conventional gender binary
Transgender woman	MTF Assigned male at birth, lives female/feminine/affirmed woman, transwoman spectrum
Transgender man	FtM Assigned female at birth, lives male, masculine, affirmed man, transmasculine spectrum
Genderqueer	New term used by individuals who do not identify as either male or female or identify as both male and female, or another nonbinary way
Transsexual	A medical term used to describe a subset of transgender individuals who have transitioned to the opposite sex

FtM, female-to-male; MTF, male-to-female.

Understand that the concepts of sexual orientation and gender identity are separate and distinct. Transgender people have a range of sexual orientations and attractions—they may identify as gay, straight, lesbian, bisexual, or none. Terms should be used to reflect their affirmed gender (and not their sex assigned at birth). See also Table 12.1.

- A trans woman who is attracted to another woman is likely a lesbian.
- A trans man attracted to other men is likely a gay man.
- A trans woman who is attracted to a man would likely consider themselves heterosexual and similar for a trans man.
- Some transgender people may identify themselves as a queer person while others may use identifiers such as nonbinary. These are people who feel that their gender cannot be encapsulated within the binary definitions of a man or women, or masculine or feminine.
  - Some nonbinary people experience gender dysphoria and some do not.

MEDICAL ISSUES FOR THE TRANS COMMUNITY

Many transgender people and advocacy groups do not consider gender variance a psychiatric disease. Instead, it is a human variation that does, in some cases, require medical attention.

Fast Facts

A patient being transgender might not hold relevance to a particular clinical encounter; however, references and acknowledgment of their gender identity in the medical record and patient encounter will enable the nurse to provide culturally competent patient-centered care.

Diagnostic and Statistical Manual of Mental Disorders, Fifth Edition

- Like homosexuality that was listed as pathological until 1973, the identities of transgender and gender nonconforming people are no longer considered a mental disorder in the *DSM-5*.
- In the new manual, transgender people may be diagnosed with gender dysphoria, which communicates and recognizes the emotional distress that can result from the incongruence between a person's experienced and expressed gender and their assigned gender.
  - This update enables transgender people to receive affirmative treatment and transition care without the stigma of a disorder.
- A concern may still arise that the presence of gender dysphoria in the *DSM-5* will even allow the diagnosis to pathologize.
- Although many people who have navigated their transition to a place of satisfaction and self-comfort may no longer experience "undue distress" that is consistent with the diagnosis of gender dysphoria, it is still likely needed in our current health system to allow for long-term access to care and receive insurance benefits related to hormonal and other care.

Diagnostic Criteria for Gender Dysphoria According to the Diagnostic and Statistical Manual of Mental Disorders, Fifth Edition

An individual who is diagnosed with gender dysphoria must have experienced at least two of the following for at least 6 months:

1. A marked incongruence between one's experienced/expressed gender and primary and/or secondary sex characteristics (or the anticipated secondary sex characteristics in young adolescents).
2. Any of the following as a strong desire:
   a. To be rid of one's primary and/or secondary sex characteristics because of a marked incongruence with one's experienced/expressed gender (or a desire to prevent the development of the anticipated secondary sex characteristics in young adolescents)
   b. For the primary and/or secondary sex characteristics of another gender
   c. To be of a gender different from one's assigned gender
   d. To be treated as a gender different from one's assigned gender
   e. A strong conviction that one has the typical feelings and reactions of a gender different from one's assigned gender
3. The condition is associated with distress or impairment in social, occupational, or other important areas of functioning that are clinically significant (adapted from the *DSM-5*).

COMMON CARE AND TREATMENTS OF TRANSGENDER PEOPLE

- Hormone therapy
- Preoperative medical screenings
- Postoperative care
- Management of surgical complications
- Routine health assessments and care
- Cancer care and screenings
  - Ensure that transgender patients receive cancer education and screenings respective of their natal (birth) sex:
    - Breast cancer screenings for transgender men who still have breasts or residual breast tissue, familial history
    - Prostate examinations for transgender women
- Reproductive health
  - Contraception
  - Family planning
  - STD/HIV testing and counseling
- Health promotion
- Management of other chronic medical illnesses unrelated to their gender identity or transition (Table 12.2)

Table 12.2

Common Transition-Related Surgical Procedures	
Male to Female	**Female to Male**
Vaginoplasty	Mastectomy
Orchiectomy	Hysterectomy
Breast augmentation	Oophorectomy
Facial feminization	Vaginectomy
Adam's apple removal/reduction thyrochondroplasty	Scrotoplasty
	Phalloplasty
Liposuction	Metoidioplasty
Body contouring	(clitoral reconstruction)

BEHAVIORAL HEALTH ISSUES FOR THE TRANS COMMUNITY

- Exploration of gender identity
- Assistance and support in coming out and transitioning
- Mood and behavioral conditions that may arise from stressors of living as a transgender person
- Care for mental health issues that may occur that are unrelated to gender or their transgender experience
- Depression and anxiety
- Substance use

HEALTH DISPARITIES, HEALTH RISKS, AND BARRIERS TO CARE

Transgender people face many barriers to culturally competent and affirming healthcare. These barriers further perpetuate the health disparities faced by this population. Most of these barriers stem from the lack of knowledgeable and trained healthcare providers in transgender health.

Nurses play an essential role in improving the health and access to healthcare of transgender people by educating themselves about transgender health. By understanding the sociocultural, institutional, and financial barriers that face transgender people, nurses are better equipped to help dismantle those barriers and provide culturally competent care to this population.

When compared to the general population, transgender people see higher rates of the following (Levitt, 2015):

- Physical violence (26%)
- Sexual assault (10%–14%)

- Attempted suicide (30%–64%)
- Substance use (36%–53%)
- Depression (40%–50%)
- Anxiety (47%)

Many transgender people face different forms of adversity that can negatively impact their mental health. Nurses and providers need to understand the adverse actions that transgender people face related to their gender identity:

- Family rejection
- Verbally harassed or disrespected in a public venue (such as hotel, restaurant)
- Harassed when presenting ID
- Loss of job or housing

The most significant barrier that transgender people face in healthcare is the lack of providers who are knowledgeable and trained in healthcare. A study completed by the Williams Institute at UCLA showed that access to gender-affirming medical care is associated with a lower prevalence of suicidal thoughts and attempts:

- Approximately 91% of transgender respondents have had lifetime suicide thoughts after being refused treatment by a healthcare provider.
- 59.5% of respondents attempted suicide after being refused by a provider in the last year (James et al., 2016).

Fast Facts

Transgender people face unique health disparities and barriers to healthcare, with the most significant being a lack of culturally competent healthcare providers. Nurses play a crucial role in reducing these disparities by educating themselves about transgender health.

Transgender people can face other barriers when accessing healthcare and health services:

- Harassment, misgendering, and objectification when seeking healthcare.
  - These barriers lead to transgender people avoiding or delaying healthcare.

- Patient fear and mistrust.
  - Stemming from minority stress, transgender people face high levels of psychological stress from stigma and discrimination. This leaves many wondering, "Will I be treated?"
- Inconsistency in treatment availability.
  - A lack of culturally competent providers or providers willing to treat transgender people can lead to long wait times and variability in treatment in practices.
  - Transgender people in rural areas may not have immediate access to trained providers.
  - Providers who are not trans competent may be unwilling to prescribe hormones or other referrals, which can lead to transgender people obtaining hormone or silicone injections in unconventional ways that place them at a higher risk of injury, infection, or death.
- Financial and insurance barriers
  - Many transgender people lack insurance coverage, which may be in part to the higher prevalence of unemployment and poverty among the transgender population. This phenomenon is likely contributed to the history of employment discrimination in the United States.
  - Private insurers have historically excluded gender-affirming treatments.
    - The Affordable Care Act made provisions that it was illegal for any health program, insurer, or organization that receives federal funds to discriminate; however, it was never clear if gender identity was a protected class.
    - In 2020, the Supreme Court made a historic ruling that expanded employment discrimination protections to include gender identity and sexual orientation under the landmark Civil Rights Act. The impact of this ruling on healthcare is yet to be determined but has the potential to improve the health and well-being of transgender people drastically.
  - The lack of trans-competent healthcare providers can also lead to transgender people paying out of pocket for providers who may be outside of their health plan.
  - Nurses play a significant role in protecting transgender health by understanding local and federal laws regarding gender identity discrimination and helping transgender people navigate their healthcare insurer.
    - Assisting transgender patients with prior authorizations or contacting their insurer about applicable co-pays, coverage options, and out-of-pocket expenses.

NURSING CONSIDERATIONS

- Create a welcoming environment for transgender patients by understanding that they may have experienced many barriers accessing healthcare.
- Ask patients what name they would like to be called and their pronouns.
- Create intake forms that ask about sexual orientation, gender identity, and their name/pronoun.
- Do not out patients without their permission.
- Provide transgender, qualified healthcare referrals.
- Provide transgender, sensitive, and informed patient education materials.
- Explicitly include gender identity and expression in all nondiscrimination policies.
- Ensure that transgender patients can use the bathroom that matches their gender identity or the use of gender-neutral bathrooms.
- Only ask questions that are related to the patient's healthcare.
- Ask patients what language or terms they would like to use for their bodies.
- Provide training for all staff members on transgender health and communication.
- Continue education for nursing and other healthcare providers on current transgender health protocols and standards of care.

Fast Facts

Culturally competent communication is vital to the nurse–patient relationship when interacting with transgender patients. Treating them as an individual and recognizing them as a person is critical.

CASE STUDY

A 32-year-old woman presents to the ED complaining of tooth pain. She tells the receptionist that she has not seen a dentist or doctor for over 10 years, and she is worried about a tooth infection. On her intake form, she reports that her current gender identity is female, and her sex assigned at birth was male. Her first name is Angela, but her identification lists her first name as Andrew. While she is waiting to see a

(continued)

(continued)

physician, she enters the women's restroom. Another patient comes out of the women's restroom and reports to the receptionist that she thinks a man is using the women's restroom. The receptionist sends a patient care technician into the women's restroom to see if there is a problem. The technician returns and says everything is all right. Angela exits the restroom and sits in the waiting area. A nurse appears with a chart and calls for Andrew. Angela avoids looking at the nurse.

The nurse repeatedly calls for Andrew. The patient who had reported a man in the women's room laughs derisively. Eventually, Angela gets up and goes to the nurse, and on her way to the door, Angela hears the patient who had reported a man in the women's room commenting, "I knew it was a man." The nurse says to Angela, "You must be Andrew? Come with me." Angela is quickly roomed and anxiously awaits to be seen by the physician and contemplates leaving the ED. The physician enters the room, introduces herself, and then asks, "So Angela, what brings you in tonight?"

1. How would you have handled the restroom complaint by the other patient in the ED?
   a. In this example, the receptionist and the tech handled the situation appropriately. They addressed the concern of the other patient while respecting the gender identity of Angela. At the institution level, the creation of gender-neutral bathrooms can help prevent this situation from occurring by removing gender from the equation when patients are using restroom facilities.
2. What is the best way for nursing and other staff to address the patient's when their names do not match their identification documents?
   a. In this scenario, Angela provided both names to the receptionist. Nurses and healthcare organizations must honor and recognize the chosen names of transgender individuals, even if it does not match their ID. For patient safety and billing purposes, there may be times where the name of their state ID must be used. Still, by documenting their chosen name visibly, nurses and healthcare providers can create an inclusive and welcoming healthcare experience. The use of their chosen name can further validate their identity.
   b. If Angela's name was documented on the form the nurse was reading from, then when Angela approached the nurse, the nurse should have used her preferred name—both when calling for the patient and in greeting. By further using the name Andrew, the nurse is invalidating Angela's gender identity. This can leave the patient with feelings of mistrust and anxiety. When the physician used Angela's name, it can help erase feelings of anxiety or worry.

c. *If Angela's name was not listed on the form, the nurse should have responded as such "Hello, I see that it has Andrew listed as your name. Do you have another name that you would wish for us to call you? I'm sorry that I used the wrong name—we are working on updating our system so that we can better care for you." The nurse should validate to Angela that she respects her name and that she will work to make sure that Angela knows she is respected, and her care is essential to the nurse and the organization.*

3. *How should the nurse or receptionist have handled the patient who harassed Angela as she was leaving the waiting room?*
   a. *This would depend on organizational policies, but it is essential to stress the nondiscrimination policy and code of conduct that are in place. All people, regardless of gender identity, should be able to receive healthcare and services without harassment from other patients or staff. Furthermore, the nurse or receptionist should apologize to Angela about the experience and how they will work together to create a better experience for Angela in the future.*

Further Reading

American Psychiatric Association. (2013). *Diagnostic and statistical manual of mental disorders* (5th ed.). https://doi.org/10.1176/appi.books.9780890425596

American Psychological Association. (n.d.). *Answers to your questions about transgender people, gender identity, and gender expression.* https://www.apa.org/topics/lgbt/transgender

Hein, L. C., & Levitt, N. (2014). Caring for...Transgender patients. *Nursing Made Incredibly Easy!, 12*(6), 28–36. https://doi.org/10.1097/01.nme.0000454745.49841.76

James, S. E., Herman, J. L., Rankin, S., Keisling, M., Mottet, L., & Anafi, M. (2016). *The report of the 2015 U.S. Transgender Survey.* National Center for Transgender Equality.

Lamba Legal. (2016). *Transgender affirming hospital policies.* https://www.lambdalegal.org/sites/default/files/publications/downloads/fs_20160525_transgender-affirming-hospital-policies.pdf

Levitt, N. (2015). Clinical nursing care for transgender patients with cancer. *Clinical Journal of Oncology Nursing, 19*(3), 362–366. https://doi.org/10.1188/15.CJON.362-366

World Professional Association for Transgender Health. (n.d.). *Standards of care version 7.* Retrieved January 17, 2021, from https://www.wpath.org/publications/soc

13

Understanding Hormone Therapy

Hormone therapy is a medical treatment process for people who are seeking to change their physical bodies to match their gender identity. Hormone replacement therapy (HRT) is one of the many ways that a transgender person can transition during their gender affirmation process. This chapter will provide the nurse with the basics of hormone therapy and the implications for nursing care.

In this chapter, you will learn:

1. The basics of hormone therapy
2. Common female to male therapies
3. Common male to female therapies
4. Nursing considerations for patients receiving hormone therapy

TRANSGENDER HORMONE THERAPY

- The purpose of hormone therapy is to provide exogenous endocrine hormones to induce either feminizing or masculinizing changes in a person.
- Hormone therapy is considered a medically necessary intervention for many transgender individuals.
- As with any medications, HRT should be monitored for desired results, side effects, and long-term management.

- Nurses need to have a basic understanding of HRT because they may be called upon to administering the medications, provide patient education, and monitor for side effects and desired results.
- Hormone therapy is highly individualized for transgender people.
- Some may seek a more androgynous presentation, while others may desire more masculinization or feminization.
- It is estimated that 75% of transgender people take hormones.
- The use of HRT is considered gender affirming.
- Some patients may be receiving hormone therapy by prescription or through other means (e.g., purchased over the internet).
- Many studies have proven an increase in quality of life and psychological adjustment among transgender people on hormonal therapy before surgery.
- Prescribers of hormonal therapy can be of varying specialties:
  - Endocrinology, family medicine, internal medicine, obstetrics and gynecology, and psychiatry
- There are no specific training certifications for providing hormone therapy.
- Effects usually take over 2 years, but timing can be variable.

Fast Facts

Hormone therapy plays a vital role in the health and well-being of transgender people.

Criteria for Hormone Therapy

- Persistent, well-documented gender dysphoria as per the *Diagnostic and Statistical Manual of Mental Health*, Fifth Edition (*DSM-5*)
- Capacity to make a fully informed decision and to consent for treatment
- Age of consent in a given country
- If significant medical or mental health concerns are present, they must be reasonably well controlled.

HORMONAL THERAPY FOR MALE-TO-FEMALE TRANSGENDER PATIENTS

- Estrogen is the hormone of choice for male-to-female (MTF) to transgender patients.
- Estrogen is available in oral, injection, and transdermal forms.

- Estrogen therapy lowers serum testosterone levels and raises serum estradiol levels.
- A combination of estrogen and "antiandrogens" is the most commonly studied regimen for feminization.
- Androgen-reducing medications, from a variety of classes of drugs, have the effect of reducing either endogenous testosterone levels or testosterone activity, and thus diminishing masculine characteristics such as body hair.
- Educate patients that some effects of hormone therapy, such as breast enlargement and decreased sperm production, are permanent.

Fast Facts

Estrogen significantly increases the risk of venous thromboembolism (VTE) in transgender women.

Potential Adverse Effects of Estrogen

- Estrogen appears to increase the risk of VTE
- Elevation in blood pressure
- Migraines

Estrogen Therapy Results

- Breast development
- Redistribution of body fat
- Reduction of body hair
- Stopping of scalp hair loss
- Softening of the skin
- Testicular degeneration and loss of erections
- Reduction of upper body strength

Antiandrogens

- Spironolactone, bicalutamide, flutamide, finasteride, and others.
- Commonly used in trans women who have not had an orchiectomy.
- Blocks the effects of testosterone.
- Allows estrogen to develop typical female secondary sex characteristics.
- Finasteride targets dihydrotestosterone (DHT), not testosterone.
  - Not as effective at lowering total testosterone levels.

- Spironolactone, an antihypertensive agent, directly inhibits testosterone secretion and androgen binding to the androgen receptor.
    - Blood pressure and electrolytes need to be monitored because of the potential for hyperkalemia.
- Cyproterone acetate is a progestational compound with antiandrogenic properties.
    - This medication is not approved in the United States because of concerns over potential hepatotoxicity, but it is used in other countries.
- GnRH agonists (e.g., Lupron) are neurohormones that block the gonadotropin-releasing hormone receptor, thus blocking the release of follicle-stimulating hormone and luteinizing hormone. This leads to a highly effective gonadal blockade.
    - These medications are expensive and may not be covered by insurance.
    - Only available as injectables or implants.

REGIMENS FOR MASCULINIZING HORMONE THERAPY

- Testosterone is the hormone of choice for the treatment of female-to-male (FTM) patients.
    - Testosterone generally can be given orally, transdermally, or parenterally (IM), although buccal and implantable preparations are also available.
- Many of the changes in testosterone therapy are permanent.
    - Increased facial and body hair.
    - Clitoral enlargement.
    - Deepened voice.
    - Male-patterned baldness.
- Finasteride can also be used to prevent male-patterned baldness in transgender men.
    - Likely slow or decrease secondary hair growth.
    - May slow or decrease clitoromegaly as well.

Fast Facts

Some effects of hormone therapy are reversible, while others may be permanent.

Risks of Testosterone Therapy

- Hepatoxicity
- Increased risk of sleep apnea
- Lower HDL cholesterol
- Polycythemia
- Insulin resistance
- Elevated triglycerides
- Unknown effects on breast, endometrial, and ovarian tissues

Physical Effects of Female-to-Male Hormone Therapy

- Deepened voice
- Clitoral enlargement (variable)
- Growth in facial and body hair
- Cessation of menses
- Atrophy of breast tissue
- Decreased percentage of body fat compared to muscle mass

NURSING CONSIDERATIONS FOR ALL PATIENTS RECEIVING HORMONAL THERAPY

- Assess patient's well-being with the transition.
- Assess the social effect of transition.
- Assess the progression and the degree of masculinization or feminization.
- Monitor mood cycles and adjust medication as indicated.
- Discuss any family issues.
- Review medication use.
- Keep the surgical sites clean and assess for signs/symptoms of infection.
- Monitor function of genitals.
- Encourage healthcare maintenance.
  - Pap smear, breast examination, mammogram, STD screening, and prostate screening.
- Counsel regarding sexual activity.
- Teach MTF patients that they can still get their opposite-sex partners pregnant.
  - To make enough sperm, patients should stop taking feminizing hormones for at least 3 to 6 months.
  - FTM patients can get pregnant whether they are taking hormones or not if they still have their reproductive organs.

- Teach transgender patients to use birth control without hormones.
- Advise the patients to be aware that unprotected sex not only leads to unwanted pregnancies but also puts them at risk for STDs.

CASE STUDY

Kristia is a transgender female who is seeing a nurse practitioner (NP) at a local health center for the first time in about 5 years. Her legal name is Karl. Kristia has not been to a primary care office because she has had negative encounters with nurses and doctors. She has a general distrust of healthcare professionals because she feels that they purposely misgender her and do not care about transgender health. Kristia is in a long-term relationship and recently married a cisgender male. Kristia's partner, Steven, is a patient at this health center and has told her about his positive experiences and the need for Kristia to establish care.

When entering the room, the NP initially pauses as they expected to see a patient named Karl. However, Kristia is clearly presenting as female. Kristia notices this pause and becomes visibly frustrated. The NP, noticing this change, introduces themselves and attempts to salvage the relationship by asking Kristia about her preferred name and pronouns. Kristia responds and appears to relax.

During the patient interview, Kristia reveals to the NP that she has been purchasing injectable estrogen from the internet for the last 2 years. She has not seen any provider during this time. Kristia is happy with the outcomes of the estrogen but does mention that the cost can sometimes be a barrier.

In this clinical situation, what questions and concerns should the NP ask and address with Kristia?

1. *The NP should further assess the integrity of estrogen that Kristia is purchasing online.*

   a. *What is the website?*
   b. *What is the packaging of the product?*

If amenable, the NP should ask Kristia to bring the product to her next visit. The NP should also inquire about where Kristia is getting the syringes and needles, how does she use those, and if she uses anyone else's or shares hers with other people.

   a. *Does she use new needles each time that she injects?*
   b. *Where and how does she inject?*

Depending on these answers, the NP should provide education as well as screenings such as hepatitis C and HIV.

2. *The NP should complete a thorough physical examination, including weight, height, and blood pressure. The need for breast, genital, and rectal examinations, which are sensitive issues for most transsexual, transgender, and gender-nonconforming patients, should be based on individual risks and preventive healthcare needs. The NP should establish baseline laboratory values to assess initial risk and evaluate possible future adverse events.*

3. *Monitoring for adverse events should include both clinical and laboratory evaluation.*

   a. *Follow-up should include:*
      i. *Careful assessment for signs of cardiovascular impairment and VTE through measurement of blood pressure*
      ii. *Weight and pulse*
      iii. *Heart and lung examinations*
      iv. *Examination of the extremities for peripheral edema, localized swelling, or pain*

Laboratory monitoring should be based on the risks of hormone therapy, Kristia's individual comorbidities and risk factors, and the specific hormone regimen itself.

4. *The NP should consider providing a limited (1–6 months) prescription for hormones while helping patients find a provider who can prescribe long-term hormone therapy. (This is known as bridging.) The NP should further assess Kristia's current regimen for safety and drug interactions and substitute safer medications or doses when indicated. During the assessment, the NP must ask Kristia if she has ever had a psychosocial assessment and refer her to a qualified mental health professional if appropriate and feasible. It is important that if the NP decides to prescribe bridging hormones, they must establish limits as to the duration of bridging therapy—typically 1 to 6 months.*

Further Reading

Mayer, K. H., Potter, J., Goldhammer, H., & Makadon, H. J. (2015). *The Fenway guide to lesbian, gay, bisexual, and transgender health*. American College of Physicians.

World Professional Association for Transgender Health. (2011). *Standards of care version 7*. https://www.wpath.org/publications/soc

14

Caring for LGBTQ Youth

LGBTQ youth, like their heterosexual and gender normative peers, are in a critical stage of growth and development. The health needs of LGBTQ youth and adolescents should be viewed within the context of general health and development. This chapter will help the under to understand the unique issues and health risks that frequently affect LGBTQ adolescents and how the nurse can best care for and support LGBTQ youth during this critical development stage of their lives.

In this chapter, you will learn:

1. Unique health needs and concerns of LGBTQ youth
2. How to engage with LGBTQ youth about their health
3. Care considerations for improving nursing care of LGBTQ youth

INTRODUCTION

During adolescence and young adulthood, people start to explore and construct their own unique identities. For some, this may be when they recognize that they are LGBTQ. Various age ranges can describe this population, but the standard range is 13 to 24 years old (Trevor Project, 2020).

LGBTQ youth are primarily dependent on their family and peers for guidance and economic support. Some youth may fear that their family or friends will not accept their sexual orientation or gender identity. This can pose significant psychological stressors and negatively impact their health and well-being.

Although this group will undergo the same developmental milestones as their heterosexual and cisgender counterparts, LGBTQ young adults may experience stigma, discrimination, and societal/familiar disapproval of their sexual or gender identity. This may result in LGBTQ adolescents feeling isolated or marginalized and lead to an internalization of shame or hatred.

An online survey of 10,000 adolescents found that non-LGBTQ youth listed grades, college, and career as their top three concerns. LGBTQ youth reported nonaccepting families, school/bullying problems, and fear of being outed as their top concerns (HRC, 2020). See Box 14.1.

BOX 14.1 LGBTQ YOUTH BY THE NUMBERS

- Under 50% of LGBTQ respondents disclosed their sexual orientation at school. Data shows that LGBTQ youth are less likely to disclose their gender identity than sexual orientation.
- Youth who have experienced conversion therapy are twice as likely to attempt suicide compared to those who did not.
- About two-thirds of LGBTQ youth report that they have experienced challenges to their sexual identity.
- Upward of 39% of LGBTQ considered suicide in the past year.
- More than half (58%) of transgender and nonbinary youth have experienced questioning or harassment when attempting to use a bathroom that corresponds to their gender identity.
- Many LGBTQ youth (71%) report feelings of sadness or hopelessness that lasted for at least 2 weeks.
- LGBTQ youth reported high rates (71%) of discrimination because of their gender identity or sexual orientation.
- 98% of surveyed LGBTQ youth felt that safe spaces and social networking sites are especially valuable and important.
- LGBTQ youth reported that a crisis intervention organization that focuses on LGBTQ youth is an important resource for them.

Source: The Trevor Project. (2020). *The Trevor Project national survey*. https://www.thetrevorproject.org/survey-2021/

In comparison to general youth, LGBTQ youth are at a higher risk of:

- Suicide attempts
- Bullying victimization
- Substance abuse
- Homelessness (due to family rejection)
- Sexual risk behaviors

NURSING CONSIDERATIONS FOR LGBTQ YOUTH

Despite the grim picture this information may portray, most LGBTQ youth overcome these challenges and lead healthy, well-adjusted lives. Nurses and healthcare providers are well equipped to assist LGBTQ youth struggling with sexual or gender identity issues. Nurses have the opportunity to help make this developmental stage a time of healthy discovery and self-acceptance.

Create a welcoming clinical environment and learn how to provide culturally competent care to LGBTQ youth. Develop the skills to ask questions in a nonjudgmental way about sexuality, sexual orientation, and gender identity. Treat the social and psychological stressors that LGBTQ youth may face surrounding their sexuality and gender identity with the same attention as physical ailments.

The nursing care of LGBTQ youth should promote healthy development, social and emotional well-being, and physical wellness while understanding the impact that their emerging sexuality and gender identity may have on those domains.

LGBTQ YOUTH HEALTH CONCERNS

Sexual Health

- LGBTQ youth may hide their sexual health concerns because of fear, shame, or embarrassment.
- Normalize the discussion of sexual health with an open tone of voice.
- Ask straightforward questions.
- Avoid making assumptions about who and who is not having sex.
    - For example, do not assume that the "honors student" is not having sex or that all LGBTQ adolescents have had a sexual encounter.
- Ask to follow-up questions to assess for risks accurately.
- Explore their use of condoms, frequency, and provide counseling about safer sex practices.

Mental Health

- Additional stress can be created by the need to manage sexual or gender identity.
- Adolescence can be when mental health issues such as depression, anxiety, psychosis, and bipolar symptoms may occur.
- "Coming out" or beginning to experiment with same-sex encounters may cause youth to have internal psychological conflict or conflict with family and friends.
- Other psychological stressors
  - New schools or peer groups
  - Entering college
  - Independent living
  - Finding employment
- Suicide
  - The leading cause of death among U.S. adolescents, and some research has shown that it might be the leading cause of death among LGBTQ youth.
  - LGBTQ youth may be three times more likely to self-report a suicide attempt (Trevor Project, 2020).
  - Distressed patients frequently visit their providers in the days, weeks, or months preceding a successful suicide—this highlights the importance of nurses assessing for psychological safety and well-being. Prompt identification of distress can be an opportunity for early intervention.

Substance Use

- LGBTQ youth are more likely to smoke cigarettes compared to the general youth population.
- Experimentation with substances can be a part of normal development. Still, they can be misused to self-medicate underlying depression or relieve the pain of loneliness, rejection, and isolation.
- Alcohol and drug use among all adolescents, including LGBTQ, are linked to destructive behaviors and adverse outcomes.
- Marijuana is the most commonly used illicit drug in adolescence, but "club drugs" may be used by gay and bisexual men. These can be used to create a sense of euphoria, social disinhibition, and heightened sexuality (ecstasy, methamphetamine, ketamine).
- Ask questions in a direct, nonjudgmental, and unbiased way about drug use and frequency.
  - Nurses in those clinical settings should familiarize themselves with the various "street terms" for different drug types.

Safety and Violence

- Violence is a leading cause of morbidity and mortality among U.S. youth.
  - LGBTQ youth often cite personal safety as a significant concern.
  - Many LGBTQ youth experience violence directly related to their sexual orientation and gender identity.
  - LGBTQ youth report high rates of verbal abuse, threats of physical violence, and overt physical assault.
- Persistent bullying and victimization can lead to anxiety, depression, underage drug and alcohol use, and unprotected sex.
- Schools are frequent sites of bullying for LGBTQ youth.

Homelessness

- LGBTQ youth often experience homelessness due to conflict with their parents about their sexual orientation or gender identity.
- Some youth are asked or forced to leave their homes because of their identity.
- Other LGBTQ youth may voluntarily leave their home as a personal decision or to escape a situation that is considered unsafe. This could be from verbal or physical antigay harassment or parental attempts to convince them to undergo therapy "to become heterosexual." Homeless youth may trade sexual activity for food, money, drugs, or shelter.
  - This increases their risk of HIV infection and other STDs.
- Primary health screenings and recommendations are often missed with homeless youth as they may only present to seek out healthcare because of acute physical symptoms.

CLINICAL CARE OF LGBTQ YOUTH

Patient–Nurse Relationship

Quality experiences are critical for LGBTQ youth to be adherent with recommended screenings and help ease adulthood transition. The primary objective with clinical encounters of LGBTQ youth should be creating a safe, open, and honest dialogue, as they may be uncomfortable or uneasy for a myriad of reasons:

- Discomfort discussing sensitive information with parents or guardians in the room.
- They are accessing healthcare for the first time alone or without parental consent.

- Fear that the nurse or provider will "out" them and so may be reluctant to disclose their sexual orientation or gender identity.
    - For some youth, this may be detrimental if the family is not accepting and could result in homelessness or abuse.
    - The nurse can use the following phrase to assist with interviewing the adolescent without a parent or guardian in the examination room:
        - "We are going to spend one time today talking together about Max's health. We will address any questions you or he may have, and then we will also spend some time with Max alone. At the end of the visit, we will come back together and talk."
    - Nurses should feel empowered to reframe this in the context of adolescent self-responsibility and self-reliance if the parent or patient shows reluctance.
- LGBTQ youth may struggle with language surrounding their orientation or identity and be unsure how to discuss sexual health topics.
    - May be evasive when asked details about their health or reason for the visit.
    - The nurse must be open and welcoming to LGBTQ youth to help elicit this information. Establishing trust is crucial.
- Note, all youth, regardless of sexual orientation or gender identity, may engage in risky behaviors (even at a very young age) that negatively impact their health.
    - Nurses must remain nonjudgmental and open.

Fast Facts

It is the nurse's duty and the healthcare provider, rather than the young patient, to conduct a complete assessment and develop a healthcare plan that addresses the patient's unique needs.

Confidentiality

One of the major concerns for LGBTQ adolescents is confidentiality. Research has shown that many LGBTQ adolescents will forgo seeking necessary healthcare because they fear their parents will discover they attempted to access care related to their sexual orientation or gender identity.

- LGBTQ youth fear that their identities will be outed, whether purposeful or not.
    - Even though the nurse may make all attempts to prioritize confidentiality, other staff such as medical assistants,

receptionists, or medical staff can accidentally or purposefully disclose their identity.

- Familiarize yourself with individual state laws and statutes that govern youth's access to confidential healthcare services.
  - Each state has different statutes regarding consent and parental notification.
  - Minors are allowed to consent to treatment without parental consent under certain circumstances:
    - Family planning services
    - Treatment for STDs or HIV
    - Emergency care
- Discuss the parameters around confidentiality of healthcare services and the circumstances in which confidentiality may be broken, such as if the minor is acutely suicidal and needs treatment.

Fast Facts

Always clarify with the patient what information is fine to share with parents and inform parents and guardians about the importance of confidential care.

Barriers to Accessing Care

- LGBTQ youth may fear that their sexual or gender identity may be disclosed inadvertently when using their parents' insurance to cover a visit.
- Many insurances will send an "Explanation of Benefits" after a healthcare encounter, impacting the youth's desire to keep the visit anonymous.
- Culturally competent care for LGBTQ youth is difficult to find as there is a lack of LGBTQ-friendly providers who focus on this population.
- LGBTQ youth who wish to maintain anonymity about their identities may seek care in public health clinics, organizations that cater to the uninsured, and/or other medical settings to anonymize.
  - This can make health screenings, vaccinations, and other care difficult as youth may seek various providers instead of a consistent provider.
- LGBTQ youth also face a disproportionate amount of socioeconomic factors that make accessing healthcare difficult:
  - Homelessness, unemployment, and lack of transportation.

Patient Interview

Often with adolescents, the chief medical complaint is usually not the primary cause for the visit. The nurse should be prepared to investigate further into potential areas of concern. Even if the youth are presenting with acne or cold symptoms, the nurse should always ask: Do you have any other problems, have any questions, or want anything else checked out while you're here? (Mayer et al., 2015).

Disclosing Sexual Orientation and Gender Identity

The goal of disclosing sexual orientation and gender identity is to create an inclusive environment for all adolescents to have the ability to ask questions, seek out help and support, and comfortably obtain healthcare and medical services. See Exhibit 14.1. Some people may not feel comfortable disclosing their sexual orientation because they have not yet entirely accepted it. Although people may identify as straight, gay, lesbian, and so forth, it is crucial to assess their sexual behaviors. As an example, some men may identify as heterosexual or straight but engage in sexual activity with other men.

Exhibit 14.1

Adolescent Patient Interview: Focus Areas and Sample Questions

- Sexual activity history
  - Do you have sex with men, women, or both?
  - There are many ways to be sexual or intimate with another person—kissing, hugging, touching, oral sex, anal sex, or vaginal sex. Have you ever had any of these experiences? Which ones? Were they with men(boys), women(girls,) or both?
- Disclosure of sexual and gender identity
  - What term (if any) do you prefer that I use to describe your sexual orientation best? Do you consider yourself gay, lesbian, bisexual, heterosexual (straight), another term, or are you not sure?
  - Have you ever talked to your parents, brothers, or sisters, or any other adult besides me about this? Any friends? What did they say?
  - It is usual for young people sometimes to be confused about their feelings and experiences. Do you have any questions that you'd like to ask me or things you would like to discuss?
- Mental health and depression
  - Over the last few weeks, have you ever felt down or depressed? Have you lost interest in doing things that you usually enjoy?

- Have you ever thought about hurting yourself? Have you ever actually tried to hurt yourself? What did you do and tell me what happened?
- Do you have a close friend or family member that is a good source of support?
- Tobacco, alcohol, and other substance use
  - Do you currently smoke cigarettes? How much and for how long? Have you ever tried to quit? Do you need help or want to stop?
  - Do you currently drink alcohol? How often? Where do you get it from, and who do you drink with?
  - Have you ever used other drugs such as marijuana, cocaine, ecstasy, GHB, crystal meth? Do you currently use any? How often? Where do you get it from?
- Safety and violence
  - Do you feel safe at home or at school?
  - How would you describe your home, school, and neighborhood in terms of support for LGBTQ people?
  - Have you ever missed school because of feeling unsafe? Has anyone ever picked on you? Was this because you are LGBTQ?
- Social media
  - Do you use social media, such as Facebook or Twitter? If so, tell me about it? (How often, what do you use it for? Are your parents aware?)
  - Do you have a cell phone? What do you use it for? Are your parents aware?
  - Where do you get your health information from?

Source: Mayer, K. H., Potter, J., Goldhammer, H., & Makadon, H. J. (2015). *The Fenway guide to lesbian, gay, bisexual, and transgender health.* American College of Physicians.

CONSIDERATIONS FOR TRANSGENDER YOUTH

- An increasing number of youth have begun to express transgender identity and at earlier ages.
- No formal protocols that have been tested by research have evaluated the use of pubertal blockers and cross-sex hormones in transgender youth.
- The nurse plays an essential role by referring the youth and family to specialists and supporting them.
- Culturally competent care is crucial at this time and can be done by maintaining respect for the person, ensuring that everyone is educated to use the correct pronouns and documentation alternate names in the medical record.

CASE STUDY

Andrea is a 15-year-old transgender patient (male to a female). Andrea and her family received education on hormonal therapy from a specialty clinic and were instructed in self-injection techniques. Andrea is coming into the office today for routine monitoring and follow-up. During the assessment, the medical assistant hears Andrea asking the nurse about her forming breasts and different bra types. On physical examination, the RN also notices bruising around the injection sites. Later in the hallway, the nurse overhears the medical assistant "I don't get why that boy was asking about wearing bras. That just seems weird."

1. What other questions and information would the nurse want to ask Andrea and her family?
   a. It would be essential to assess for side effects of the hormonal therapy and what changes or results have Andrea seen or felt as a result of the treatment.
   b. During the physical assessment, the nurse noticed bruising, which could be from poor injection technique. The nurse should review the injection administration with Andrea and her family and ask for a demonstration of the method.
   c. Using the sample questions listed before to guide the conversation, the nurse should assess mental health, safety, violence, sexual health, etc.

2. How should the RN handle the situation with the medical assistant?
   a. Provide education about the transitioning process and the importance of validating Andrea's gender identity. Andrea asking about bras shows that she is normalizing her body experience and is a typical question for female youth. The medical assistant must be educated about culturally competent care to ensure Andrea and other transgender clients' health and well-being. It would be important to know if this medical assistant's comment was from a lack of knowledge and experience or malicious intent.
   b. The nurse should also ensure that the entire office is educated about transgender youth and how to communicate.

The health needs of LGBTQ youth are much the same as the general youth population. Adolescence is a challenging time of development in which youth face various emotions and physical and sexual changes. Many LGBTQ youths meet this phase of their lives with strength and resiliency. However, this critical developmental phase of growth may be complicated by stigma and discrimination from family, friends, and society. As a result, this leads to far too many LGBTQ youths being *victims of violence, homeless, and contemplating suicide. Nurses can play a pivotal role in LGBTQ youth's lives by being aware and mindful of this population's unique health risks and issues and remember to address each patient as an individual.*

Important Care Considerations for LGBTQ Youth

- LGBTQ youth should feel safe and support in asking questions and seeking advice, support, and care.
- Discussion of confidentiality is essential and critical to the nurse–patient relationship when interacting with LGBTQ youth.
- LGBTQ youth face the same health risks and concerns as all adolescents. Stigma and discrimination associated with being LGBTQ compounds these risks and their access to care. This places them at higher risks for health disparities.
- Experimentation with drugs and alcohol can be a regular part of adolescent development. Some LGBTQ youth may use it as a way to cope with the sexual orientation or gender identity.
- Safety is a significant concern for LGBTQ youth. Many youths fear being bullied or have been bullied in their schools, neighborhoods, or families.
- Social media play an ever-increasing role in the lives of adolescents. Nurses should understand that while social media presents new opportunities for connections and communication for LGBTQ youth, it can also intimidate youth or facilitate high-risk behaviors.
- It is not the nurse's role to give specific advice about when LGBTQ youth should come out. Instead, nurses should offer support and assure the youth that they are available for assistance if needed.

Further Reading

Mayer, K. H., Potter, J., Goldhammer, H., & Makadon, H. J. (2015). *The Fenway guide to lesbian, gay, bisexual, and transgender health.* American College of Physicians.

Trevor Project. (2018, July 9). *Youth homelessness.* https://www.thetrevor project.org/get-involved/trevor-advocacy/homelessness/

Trevor Project. (2020). *The Trevor Project national survey.* https://www.thetrev orproject.org/survey-2021/

Healthy People 2030. (2021). *LGBT.* https://health.gov/healthypeople/objectives -and-data/browse-objectives/lgbt

Human Rights Campaign. (2020). *Health & aging.* https://www.hrc.org/ resources/lgbtq-youth

15

Caring for LGBTQ Older Adults

Like LGBTQ people of any age, LGBTQ older adults face health disparities related to their mental and physical health, further confounded by their age. This group of people has lived a lifetime of discrimination and stigma—living through times in the United States that were not as welcoming and progressive that our youth are living in today. This chapter will highlight the unique health needs of LGBTQ older adults and how the nurse can provide culturally competent care.

In this chapter, you will learn:

1. Unique health needs and concerns of LGBTQ older adults
2. How to engage with LGBTQ older adults about their health
3. Care considerations for improving nursing care of LGBTQ older adults

INTRODUCTION

Many LGBTQ older adults have experienced a lifetime of discrimination and stigma. Some have been forced to hide their sexual orientation or gender identity from their healthcare providers, family, employees, the government, and for some, even themselves. These older adults had lived through a time when their sexual orientation or gender identity labeled them as sinners or mentally ill. The American Psychiatric Association (APA) did not entirely remove homosexuality as a pathological disorder until 1987. For some LGBTQ older adults, this has left them with long-lasting apprehension about healthcare professionals and healthcare.

LGBTQ older adults experience the health disparities faced by all LGBTQ people with age-related health concerns. There are approximately 1 to 2 million LGBTQ older adults living in the United States (National Resource Center on LGBTQ Aging, 2018). Different age ranges can describe this population, ranging as low as 50 years old. For this book, ages 65 years and older will be generally used to define older adults.

LGBTQ older adults face physical and mental health illnesses that will be covered in this chapter, as well as other issues such as:

- Social isolation
- Depression and anxiety
- Poverty
- Chronic illnesses
- Delayed care seeking
- Poor nutrition
- Premature mortality
- Elder housing and long-term care
- Palliative care needs

SOCIAL DISPARITIES OF LGBTQ OLDER ADULTS

LGBTQ older adults face barriers to receiving proper healthcare and social support.

- LGBT older adults are more likely to be single or living alone and less likely to have children to care for them.
- Studies find LGBT older adults often rely on "families of choice" (families composed of close friends), LGBT community organizations, and affirmative religious groups for care and support.
- Financial instability and legal issues are significant concerns.
  - Disparities in earnings, employment, and discrimination can place LGBT older adults at greater financial risk.
- LGBT older adults have experienced and continue to experience discrimination due to their sexual orientation and gender identity.
  - Studies find LGBT older adults experienced high rates of lifetime discrimination and physical and verbal abuse because of their sexual and gender identity.
  - One study found that LGB seniors searching for retirement homes experienced unfavorable differential treatment (less housing availability, higher pricing, etc.) than non-LGB seniors (National Resource Center on LGBTQ Aging, 2016).

- LGBTQ people are only 20% as likely as their heterosexual counterparts to access services like senior centers and meal programs. Research has shown that older gay men or lesbians would not be welcome at 46% of local senior centers if their sexual orientation were known (LGBT Aging Center, 2021).

HEALTH ISSUES AND DISPARITIES OF LGBTQ OLDER ADULTS

Cardiovascular Health

Cardiovascular disease (CVD) is the leading cause of death for all populations in the United States. Research has found that LGBTQ people have higher rates of specific risk factors than the general population.

- Gay men have an increased recreational drug use rate, and smoking places them at a higher risk for CVD. (Mayer et al., 2015).
- Lesbian women have higher rates of obesity and smoking than the general population.
- Transgender people also have higher smoking rates than the general population, but research has also shown that sex hormones can increase CVD risk.

The nurse's role is to help modify risk factors through education, counseling, and referrals to interventions and programs.

Cancer Risk

LGBTQ older adults may have risk factors for certain cancers. Understand the risks and benefits of screenings for various cancers and create an individualized care plan for the patient.

Anal Cancer

- Caused by an infection of the human papillomavirus (HPV). Men who have sex with men (MSM) have higher rates of HPV infections when compared to the general population of men.
- Risk factors
  - Receptive anal intercourse
  - A nadir CD4 count
  - A higher HIV viral load

Cervical Cancer

- Lesbian women have significantly lower cervical screening rates when compared to heterosexual women.

- Like anal cancer, cervical cancer is caused by infection with HPV. Many lesbian women are still at risk for cervical cancer as they may have had intercourse with a man at some point in their lives.
- The U.S. Preventive Services Task Force (USPSTF) guidelines mention that most women can discontinue screening for cervical cancer at the age of 65 if they have had three consecutive negative Pap smears (USPSTF).

Prostate Cancer

- Gay and bisexual men do not have a higher incidence of prostate cancer than the general male population; however, prostate cancer is the second leading cause of cancer deaths.
- Prostate cancer can affect the sexual health of gay and bisexual men in different ways than heterosexual men.
  - The prostate gland is involved in the sexual response to receptive anal intercourse.
  - Gay and bisexual men should be counseled on sexual health implications when discussing treatment options (Mayer et al., 2015; USPSTF, 2018).

Breast Cancer

- Age is the primary risk factor for breast cancer.
  - Other risks include family history, obesity, and smoking.
- Women who have never given birth also have a higher risk of breast cancer (USPSTF, 2020).
- Current recommendations are that women aged 50 to 74 years receive biannual mammograms.

HIV-Related Cancers

- Kaposi sarcoma, lymphoma, and other cancers may be higher among older adults living with HIV (NCI, 2020).

Cancer Screening for Transgender People

- Transgender people should be educated about cancers and risk factors that correspond to their biological sex.
  - Example—transgender woman
    - A person who was born male who has transitioned to female is at risk for developing prostate cancer if the prostate was not removed.
  - Example—transgender man
    - A person who was born female who has transitioned to male may develop uterine or breast cancer if the female organs were not removed or completely removed (i.e., if residual breast tissue was left).

Fast Facts

Aging transgender people are likely to experience health problems that correspond to their biological sex and may need help coping with conditions.

Sexual Health

- Sexual function and sexual health are essential aspects of care to address when caring for LGBTQ older adults.
- Routine sexual history taking and risk-reduction counseling can greatly benefit older LGBTQ adults.
  - Screening for HIV and other STIs at routine intervals based on individual risk behaviors.

Mental Health

There is not much research on the mental health of LGBTQ older adults; however, for this population, a lifetime of managing prejudice, violence, and internalized homophobia may result in higher risks of depression, suicide, and substance abuse.

Substance Use

- Studies have shown that LGBTQ older adults are more likely to smoke and drink excessively than the general population.

Aging

- LGBTQ older adults have concerns about discrimination in healthcare, employment, and long-term care.
- One study showed that one-third of aging gay men and lesbian women identified prejudice as their top concern for aging (Mayer et al., 2015).

Isolation and Support

- LGBTQ older adults are often found with "chosen families" or a "family of choice" or without traditional family support to help them with age-related needs and care.
  - "Family of choice": A term used to describe a diverse family structure that includes close friends, partners, and/or significant others who are not biologically or legally related (SAGE, 2020).
- Studies have shown that gay and bisexual men are two times as likely to be living alone. Lesbian and bisexual women were found to be one third more likely to be living alone (Mayer et al., 2015).

- Many older LGBTQ adults do not have children.
- Family relationships may be strained or nonexistent due to the family not supporting or accepting their sexual orientation or gender identity.

Fast Facts

LGBTQ older adults are more likely to live alone and not have children. This population may rely on their "chosen families" and a network of friends for support.

- Nurses must recognize the possibility of isolation and loneliness in this population and understand the context of a "family of choice" to help support the older LGBTQ adult in decision-making and advance directives.

END OF LIFE

LGBTQ older adults can have complex needs during end of life and palliative care. Years of internalized homophobia, minority stress, and stigma can impact older LGBTQ adults' mental health during the end of life.

LGBTQ older adults may fear that disclosing their sexual orientation or gender identity near end of life could lead to discrimination or estrangement of family members.

Understand the surviving spouse or partner of an older LGBTQ adult may experience disenfranchised grief. This phenomenon occurs when a surviving spouse or partner's needs are ignored or forgotten by family, healthcare providers, and the legal systems. For example, a surviving partner may be excluded from medical decisions, funeral arrangements, and estate planning if they are not legally married.

Advance Directives

- Same-sex marriage is now the law of the land in the United States as of 2016; however, there may be some LGBTQ older adults who do not have a significant other or are not married to them.
- Advance directives are a written statement about a person's wishes regarding medical treatments, including living wills, do-not-resuscitate orders, and healthcare power of attorney.

Fast Facts

Talk to LGBTQ older adults about their advance directives. If they become incapacitated to make decisions, they can be subject to state laws that may not allow their chosen family or partners in medical decisions or visitations.

In 2011, the Department of Health and Human Services implemented a regulation that all Medicare/Medicare facilities must allow patients to decide who has visitation rights and make medical decisions for them, regardless of sexual orientation, gender identity, or family makeup.

Understand your applicable state laws when advising LGBTQ older adults about their advance directives.

CASE STUDY

Rose is a 67-year-old lesbian who lives on her own. Rose arrived at the emergency room after falling in her apartment and suffering a broken hip. Rose has surgery on her hip and is awaiting placement at a skilled nursing facility for rehabilitation. However, her discharge has been complicated because she has a history of alcohol abuse, which was a contributing factor to her fall.

When asked about her alcohol use, Rose states that she was in a heterosexual marriage for 25 years. During that time, she drank in secret to help take away the guilt that she had about the feelings she had for women. She now drinks because it helps with her feelings of loneliness—she has never been able to be in a long-term relationship with a woman after her divorce (Adapted from Rowan, 2012).

Rose asks the RN case manager if they have to tell the skilled nursing facility about Rose being a lesbian or if this is something that can be kept a secret. When pressed for more detail, Rose says that she is fearful that the staff at the facility might treat her differently if they knew.

1. *What other questions should the case manager or healthcare team ask Rose?*
   a. *It would be helpful to understand more about Rose's feelings about her sexuality and fears of going to the nursing home. The*

(continued)

(continued)

case manager can work with Rose to find a home that is LGBTQ-friendly, ask about their policies, and find more information for Rose. Many older adults just need someone to listen to their stories and validate their experiences. If the hospital staff can treat Rose with dignity and respect for her sexuality, it may help her accept herself.

   b. It might be helpful for Rose to be seen by social work and psychiatry to help her with her substance misuse, coping with her sexuality, and finding community support groups.

2. How should the RN case manager communicate to Rose about the disclosure of her sexuality?

   a. The case manager should clearly explain how a patient's personal information may be used or shared with accepting facilities and what information the facilities may ask of Rose.

   b. In this situation, it would be helpful for Rose to ask about policies on personal information at the nursing facility:

      i. For example, will all staff have access to all her files or just their own patients? Facility representatives should be as clear and forthright as possible when explaining the facility's confidentiality policy, as well as the sharing of patients' personal information, including information on sexual orientation and gender identity. Fully detailing how client information is kept confidential and private fosters a safe space and shows clients that they are respected and that they do not need to fear intrusion or harassment.

   c. It is important to remember that Rose has lived through a time full of discrimination and is working through her own sexual identity. It can be expected that she is defensive or worrisome about disclosing her identity when she is unsure how the answer may affect her care or treatment. It is the duty of the case manager and others on the care team to ensure that Rose has the opportunity to choose a facility where she feels safe and respected.

3. While in the nursing facility what are ways that nursing staff can deliver culturally competent care to Rose?

   a. It is important that the nursing staff understand that Rose may not yet be open about her sexuality in every aspect of their lives.

   b. Do not refer to Rose as "LGBTQ" or a lesbian in a public setting without first getting permission. This is particularly important in group settings such as senior centers, day programs, or support groups. While there may be many LGBTQ people who are out and have no issues being so to anyone and everyone, it is still important for staff to have Rose's permission.

c. Be supportive when and if Rose self-identifies as LGBTQ. When an LGBTQ older adult self-identifies (especially if they appear nervous or uncomfortable), it is helpful to provide supportive affirmation (e.g., "Thank you for telling me…," or "I appreciate you sharing that with me…").

d. Focus on the whole person. Sexual orientation and gender identity are just two aspects of Rose. A way to build trust with an LGBT older adult is to be sure to ask about their hobbies, social circles, and interests. While sexual orientation and gender identity are important, they should not be the sole focus of discussion.

LGBTQ older adults face the same health challenges as other aging Americans in our country, but they also have specific social, physical, and mental health needs. This population may be invisible in

BOX 15.1 COMMUNICATION TIPS AND STRATEGIES

- Nurses in all practice settings should not make assumptions about a person's sexual orientation or gender identity.
- Older adults must be asked about their sexual orientations and gender identity.
  - Do not assume and treat all patients as if they are heterosexual. This invalidates the struggles that LGBTQ older adults may have faced.
- Create an opening for LGBTQ patients to talk about their family members or support system by asking open-ended questions: Who do you consider family? Who in your life is important?
- Ensure confidentiality.
- Explain why you are asking questions and remind them that these questions are asked of everyone. Normalize the experience.
- Be sensitive to and understand that many LGBTQ older adults did not have the opportunity to get married or thought that they would live to see it.
- Ask about sexual activity and do not make assumptions based on age.
- Provide referrals to community and mental health support groups and organizations.
- Have signs, fliers, and symbols in your practice setting to signal an inclusive and LGBTQ-friendly environment.

practice settings because of difficulty disclosing their sexual orientation or gender identity. Nurses can help create inclusive environments and welcome the LGBTQ older adult into healthcare settings (see Box 15.1). While LGBTQ older adults may face the negative experiences and disparities mentioned in this chapter, it is also important to note that many older LGBTQ adults live and lead healthy lives with their families, friends, and support systems. The nurse's role is to ensure that we can provide culturally competent care and services for all LGBTQ older adults.

Further Reading

LGBT Aging Center. (2021, January 13). *The LGBTIA+ aging project*. https://fenwayhealth.org/the-fenway-institute/lgbtqia-aging-project/

Mayer, K. H., Potter, J., Goldhammer, H., & Makadon, H. J. (2015). *The Fenway guide to lesbian, gay, bisexual, and transgender health*. American College of Physicians.

National Cancer Institute. (2020). *HIV infection and cancer risk*. https://www.cancer.gov/about-cancer/causes-prevention/risk/infectious-agents/hiv-fact-sheet

National Resource Center on LGBT Aging. (2016). *Inclusive questions for older adults: A practical guide to collecting data on sexual orientation and gender identity*. https://www.lgbtagingcenter.org/resources/resource.cfm?r=601

National Resource Center on LGBT Aging. (2018, July 30). *The first and only resource center dedicated to improving the lives of LGBT older adults*. https://www.sageusa.org/what-we-do/national-resource-center-on-lgbt-aging/

Rowan, N. (2012). *Older lesbian adults and alcoholism: A case study for practitioners*. https://www.aginglifecarejournal.org/older-lesbian-adults-and-alcoholism-a-case-study-for-practitioners/

U.S. Preventative Services Task Force. (2018, May 8). *Prostate cancer: Screening*. https://www.uspreventiveservicestaskforce.org/uspstf/recommendation/prostate-cancer-screening

IV

Resources for Nurses and Healthcare Organizations

16

Creating Inclusive Environments

The care environment can impact the overall healthcare experience of LGBTQ people. All people, especially those who are LGBTQ, want healthcare environments where they feel welcomed and respected. Creating an inclusive healthcare environment is not a difficult task, nor is it an expensive one. What it does require, though, is a dedicated focus and effort on diversity and inclusivity. This chapter contains information and strategies for the nurse and healthcare organizations to build a more inclusive LGBTQ environment.

In this chapter, you will learn:

1. Strategies for creating an inclusive healthcare environment
2. The importance of welcoming and inclusive spaces for LGBTQ people
3. Understand the barriers faced by LGBTQ people when accessing healthcare services

LGBTQ people require inclusive and welcoming medical care. Imagine being a lesbian walking into an examination room full of brochures, magazines, and posters of heterosexual couples. You are given a registration form that only has the option of single or married; this question is a struggle for you because you have been in a long-term relationship with another woman. Although same-sex marriage is legal across the country, you have yet to marry. Unsure of how the nurse and provider will respond, you have an internal conflict of how and what to respond to on the form. Nurses must understand that this is not a "one-off" but is a real-life example of how LGBTQ people access healthcare and their fears. It is highly likely, and research has shown that many LGBTQ people do not feel included, welcomed, or safe to disclose their sexual orientation or gender identity to nurses or their providers.

The invisibility of LGBTQ in healthcare can have dire consequences for the health and well-being of this population. Over the last few years, many resources have become available to help healthcare organizations and individuals consider ways to create a more inclusive experience for LGBTQ people.

THE JOINT COMMISSION

The Joint Commission, a primary accrediting body in the United States, has codified two requirements specific to improving care and the environment for LGBTQ people. Without meeting these two requirements, a hospital is ineligible for accreditation by the Joint Commission. This accreditation is often a necessity for some insurance reimbursements and regulatory requirements. These requirements fall under RI.01.01.01: "The hospital respects, protects, and promotes patient rights."

- EP 28: The hospital allows a family member, friend, or other individuals to be present with the patient for emotional support during the course of the stay.
- EP 29: The hospital prohibits discrimination based on age, race, ethnicity, religion, culture, language, physical or mental disability, socioeconomic status, sex, sexual orientation, and gender identity or experience.

Fast Facts

The Joint Commission requires that organizations meet two standards in delivering care to LGBTQ—allowing them visitors of their choice and including sexual orientation and gender identity and experience in their nondiscrimination statement.

These two requirements lay the foundation for improving an LGBTQ person's experience in the hospital. Historically, organizational policies have limited visitors to immediate family, which can disenfranchise LGBTQ people who have unmarried same-sex partners or who rely primarily on friends that are not their biological family for support. The second requirement sets the expectation that LGBTQ patients are entitled to equitable care. Although these provisions are in place, nurses and organizations still have to take deliberate actions and steps toward achieving LGBTQ-inclusive environments, as outlined in the rest of this chapter.

Nondiscrimination Policies

- Sexual orientation, gender identity, and expression must be explicitly outlined in nondiscrimination policies.
- Publicly display or distribute these policies in high-profile areas and easily accessible from the organization website.
- These policies are Joint Commission Standards and are required for becoming a Healthcare Equality Index Leader.
- Have a clear and specific pathway for reporting and addressing discrimination if it occurs.
- Develop and uphold a policy ensuring equal visitation.

Care and Services

- All staff receive training on culturally affirming care for LGBTQ people.
  - Vary methods of training.
  - Update training and educational materials regularly.
  - Ensure that all new and current staff receive education on an ongoing basis.
- Specific services and programs should be offered to meet the needs of LGBTQ patients.
  - Support groups, HIV and STD screenings, prevention and treatment, and transgender health programs.
  - Provide educational programs and forums that support the health and well-being of LGBTQ people.
- Maintain and create a list of LGBTQ-welcoming referrals for various services that you do not provide.
- Registration and medical history forms must be inclusive of LGBTQ relationships, identities, and families.
  - Registration is an opportunity to set the stage for LGBTQ people to feel recognized and welcomed.
  - Does your organization include sexual orientation and gender identity on intake and admission forms?
    - If not, why?

- ❏ Research in rural and urban settings has shown that both LGBTQ and non-LGBTQ people are receptive to sexual orientation and gender identity questions.
- ▪ Many transgender people have identity cards and insurance documents that do not accurately reflect their names or pronouns during their transition. To prevent miscommunication, find space to allow them the opportunity to share their name and pronouns. All staff should be trained on how to navigate this information.
- ▪ Ensure that questions are inclusive of transgender people and diverse bodies.
  - ❏ Are there questions that contain areas that specify things like "for women only"? All patients must answer these types of questions so that crucial information is not missed or overlooked.
- ▪ Collect patient demographic data on sexual orientation and gender identity in the electronic health record.
  - ❏ This is a recommendation by the Institutes of Medicine and The Joint Commission.
  - ❏ Collecting this information can help organizations trend clinical data to improve patient satisfaction and quality of care.
  - ❏ Ensure that strong privacy protections are in place for all patients.

Physical Space

- ▪ Place brochures, posters, and/or periodicals on LGBTQ topics in waiting rooms.
- ▪ Offer single-stall (unisex) bathrooms or develop policies that allow transgender people to use bathrooms that match their gender identity.
- ▪ Think about the physical space as holistically as possible.
  - ▪ Can LGBTQ people see themselves represented there?
  - ▪ Does it feel welcoming when entering?

Fast Facts

Creating an inclusive environment for LGBTQ people involves the physical space, the electronic medical record, employee education, and senior leadership action.

Community Engagement

Engaging with the local LGBTQ community is critical to creating an inclusive and welcoming environment for LGBTQ people. If they see that nurses and other healthcare providers want to be a part of their community, they will feel this when they seek healthcare.

- Cosponsor or host LGBTQ community events.
- Recognize and celebrate LGBTQ days of observance:
  - National Coming Out Day
  - Transgender Day of Remembrance
  - World AIDS Day
- Hold focus groups to understand better the needs of the LGBTQ community in your area or gain insight on the patient experience of LGBTQ people when visiting your facility.
- Include LGBT imagery in marketing and educational materials, websites, and brochures.

LGBTQ Employees

- When an organization takes steps to provide equitable treatment for LGBTQ employees and create inclusive workspaces, all employees benefit.
- Extend benefits to unmarried same-sex partners of employees.
- Offer transgender healthcare coverage.
- Create a guidebook for staff on how to approach and communicate with a coworker who is transitioning.
- Develop a plan to address the unique needs of transgender employees.
- Have a nondiscrimination and zero-tolerance policy for LGBTQ discrimination in the workplace.
- Celebrate national LGBTQ days in the workspace.
- Engage in LGBTQ community events.
  - March in the local Pride Parade.
- Recruit and retain LGBTQ staff.
  - Having open LGBTQ people on staff creates a foundation of respect and inclusivity.
- Support an LGBTQ employee resource group (ERG).
  - An ERG can offer LGBTQ employees and allies mentoring, coaching, networking, and information on programs or topics of interest. It can also be a forum to improve employee satisfaction and patient experience.

Nurse Executives

- Leadership sets the tone for an organization's culture. LGBTQ inclusiveness must be a commitment for nurse executives.
- Senior leaders should create an LGBTQ advisory group for the organization or identify a "champion" responsible for the assessment, monitoring, and implementation of LGBTQ-focused initiatives.

Given the dynamic nature of society, the government and public policy, and other driving forces behind LGBTQ inclusion in healthcare, creating an inclusive healthcare environment for LGBTQ people will continue to be a moving target. Implementation of best practices for care delivery requires dedication from nurses and other healthcare professionals.

Fast Facts

Nurses play a crucial role in creating an inclusive environment by incorporating sexual orientation and gender identity into their patient assessments.

Beyond being an ethical imperative to provide safe and respectful care to LGBTQ people, there are various other risks such as legal action, loss of federal funding, and citation or loss of accreditation for a failure to provide an inclusive environment for LGBTQ patients. Using the strategies in this chapter, the nurse will complete a self-assessment of their nursing practice and the organization in which they work. In doing so, nurses will show LGBTQ people that they are willing to provide them with the care they need and the respect they deserve.

Further Reading

Essential Access Health. (n.d.). *Providing inclusive care for LGBTQ patients: A resource guide for clinicians.* Retrieved from http://www.essential access.org/sites/default/files/Providing-Inclusive-Care-for-LGBTQ -Patients.pdf

DHHS Office of Disease Prevention and Health Promotion. (2015). *Healthy People 2020: Lesbian, gay, bisexual, and transgender health.* https://www.healthypeople.gov/2020/topics-objectives/topic/lesbian -gay-bisexual-and-transgender-health

The Joint Commission. (2011). *Advancing effective communication, cultural competence, and patient- and family- centered care for the lesbian, gay, bisexual, and trans- gender (LGBT) community: A field guide.* LGBTFieldGuide.pdf

The National LGBTQIA+ Health Education Center. (2016). *Ten things: Creating inclusive health care environment for LGBTQ people.* https://www.lgbthealtheducation.org/publication/ten-things/

17

Advocacy, Policy, and Legal Issues for LGBTQ Populations

LGBTQ people in America face discrimination in their lives daily. Many policies to protect LGBTQ people from discrimination have been passed at the federal, state, and local levels; however, there is legislation advancing bills in our country and states that target transgender people and allow the use of religion to discriminate. The chapter explores the various legal issues surrounding LGBTQ people, including the public policy that has expanded their rights to life and healthcare in America. A fundamental tenet of nursing practice is to advocate for the patient, and this chapter will help the nurse advocate for LGBTQ people at the bedside and beyond.

In this chapter, you will learn:

1. The background and significance of health policy and legislation surrounding LGBTQ people and health
2. How policy and law impact LGBTQ people and their access to healthcare
3. The importance of the Affordable Care Act (ACA) in reducing health disparities faced by LGBTQ people and improving access to care
4. Why nurses can play a key role in improving the health and well-being of LGBTQ people through policy, law, and advocacy

LGBTQ people in the United States live in almost every county and are racially and ethnically diverse. Like others, LGBTQ people in the United States want to provide for their families, pursue a life of happiness, and fully participate in the American Dream.

HISTORIC LGBTQ LEGISLATION

- LGBTQ people lacked access to marriage until 2015 when a landmark Supreme Court ruling made same-sex marriage the law of the land.
  - However, some efforts are being made to undermine these legal protections for same-sex marriages at the state level.
- Older LGBTQ adults living today experienced a time when homosexual acts and same-sex marriage were illegal. It was not until 2004 that the Supreme Court struck down sodomy laws.
- In 2020, the Supreme Court prohibited employment discrimination against LGBTQ employees.
  - While this ruling extended to employers, LGBTQ people still face the risk of discrimination in housing, education, transportation, credit, and in the jury system.
    - Only 24 states, the District of Columbia, Puerto Rico, Guam, and approximately 140 cities and counties in the United States have enacted bans on discrimination based on sexual orientation and/or gender identity.
    - This means that LGBTQ people can be denied housing and evicted or refused other services in individual states.

LGBTQ FAMILIES

Nurses working with children of LGBTQ families and planning families have to be familiar with local and federal laws. Although same-sex marriage is legal across the United States, same-sex couples can still face barriers in family planning and raising their children. Recent data shows that approximately 114,000 same-sex couples are raising children in the United States, and this number is expected to continue to grow (Williams Institute, 2020).

- The legal implications for LGBTQ families vary across the United States. With a few options, the authority to decide what constitutes a family resides mostly within state and local law.
- LGBTQ families have long faced discrimination when seeking legal parentage.

- Same-sex couples have faced legislative bans on lesbian and gay foster and adoptive parenting.
- Stereotypes and beliefs about LGBTQ people continue to threaten the ability of LGBTQ people to engage in foster and adoptive parenting.
- State-based religious freedom bills threaten LGBTQ adoptive parenting.
  - These bills enable adoption agencies to refuse to place children with LGBTQ people if doing so violates agencies' sincerely held religious beliefs. These bills can continue to stigmatize LGBTQ families and serve as a significant barrier to the right to parent for LGBTQ people.
- LGBTQ families can also face legal parenting barriers when children are conceived naturally or through other family planning methods.
  - Same-sex couples are more likely than heterosexual couples to raise nonbiological children and children produced through surrogacy and assisted reproductive technology.
  - Many states in the United States still ban or place limits on surrogacy contracts. This restricts the opportunities available for gay couples and LGBTQ families that cannot reproduce through other assisted reproductive technologies to become legal parents.
- Many states and other countries still determine parental rights make based on who is the biological parent.
  - It is advised that nonbiological parents in a same-sex relationship adopt the children of the marriage, even if a state allows both same-sex parents to be listed on a child's birth certificate.

LGBTQ CAREGIVERS

Unlike heterosexual older adults who may have robust family support, LGBTQ often turns to their "family of choice" during times of need and for caregiving. Chosen families are not legally recognized and can be contested by the biological family of an LGBTQ person. It is essential for nurses working with LGBTQ people who have caregivers that are not part of their family to educate them about advance directives and legal ramifications within your state. Incapacity can strike at any time, and we must ensure that our patients have the person who cares for them the most, making decisions during these times. Many of these documents are state specific, so it is essential to understand the applicable laws and regulations within your state. Nurses should be familiar with the following three documents:

Will

- A legal document that allows a person to designate who will receive their property when they die, how and when they will receive it. If no will is executed before the person dies, the laws of intestacy in which they reside will take effect. A will is only effective when a person dies.
- This document is for after death.

Durable Power of Attorney

- This document will ensure that if a person becomes legally incapacitated, a designated person will have the legal authority to manage all property and financial affairs.

Advance Healthcare Directive

- A document that ensures that all healthcare needs and wishes are carried out and monitored by a trusted person when they can no longer make those decisions or communicate them to healthcare providers. This document contains the instructions regarding a patient's wishes and desires for healthcare, including what end-of-life treatment is and is not desired, such as intubation, ventilators, or hydration.
- Other forms for healthcare include a living will, do not resuscitate (DNR) order, and Physician Orders for Life-Sustaining Treatment (POLST).

Fast Facts

Nurses can help ensure that LGBTQ caregivers are protected by having discussions about advance directives, wills, and durable power of attorneys.

HEALTHCARE ACCESS AND HEALTH COVERAGE

Affordable Care Act

The ACA makes far-reaching changes in health coverage and delivery of care for millions, including LGBTQ individuals. LGBTQ populations were impacted in three major areas:

1. Access to coverage and insurance market reforms
2. "Nondiscrimination" protections
3. Requirements for data collection and research

Affordable Care Act by the Numbers

- Since the ACA's implementation, uninsured rates decreased significantly among LGB adults
  - Rates dropped from 19% in 2013 to 10% in 2016, representing an estimated 369,000 fewer uninsured LGB individuals (Kates et al., 2018).
- Medicaid coverage for LGBT people in the United States increased.
  - Rates rose from 7% to 15% during the same period, representing an estimated 511,000 more LGBT individuals with Medicaid coverage.
  - These coverage changes were similar to those seen in the heterosexual population (Kates et al., 2018).

At the time of publication, the Trump Administration's recent actions have sought to scale back some of these gains; however, with changing administrations, the future of ACA is uncertain.

Fast Facts

The ACA helped increase healthcare accessibility to hundreds of thousands of underinsured LGBTQ people. The ACA also improved healthcare access through nondiscrimination policies and sexual orientation and gender identity data collection.

Data Collection

The ACA calls for the inclusion of systematic data collection and surveillance on health disparities, which many groups have recognized as LGBTQ populations.

Nondiscrimination Protections

In addition to expanding healthcare coverage to LGBTQ people, the ACA also extended new healthcare protections.

- ACA Section 1557 prohibits discrimination on the basis of existing civil rights law by any entity taking money from the U.S. government. This includes any hospital or healthcare organization that is receiving Medicaid or Medicare funding.
- In 2012, a federal regulation outlawed sexual orientation and gender identity discrimination by qualified health plans traded on state health insurance marketplaces.
  - However, it is essential to note that although this regulation protects against insurance discrimination, it does not apply to healthcare discrimination.

- More than half of Americans are employed through their employer. This is regulated by the Employee Retirement Income Security Act, which does not prohibit sexual orientation and gender identity discrimination.
- Like the ones built into the ACA, nondiscrimination protections are important to LGBTQ people because they offer another layer of protection for this vulnerable community. Many protections do not exist.

LGBTQ People and Health Coverage

- Research finds bisexual individuals have more limited access to care while lesbian and gay individuals have rates comparable to heterosexual adults.
  - Bisexual adults did not have routine medical care and often forwent medical care due to cost.
- Almost 4 in 10 LGBTQ people living in poverty have medical debt, and more than 4 in 10 have reported postponing medical care due to costs (Kates et al., 2018).
- In 2017, many large-scale employers (greater than 1,000 employees) offered same-sex couples the same health benefits as opposite-sex couples.
  - However, fewer than two-thirds (64%) of employees at the smallest employers (between 3 and 49 employees) have access to those same benefits (Kates et al., 2018).
- As of January 2014, individuals can no longer be denied most private market insurance due to a preexisting condition, such as HIV, mental illness, or a transgender medical history.
- Health plans are now required to cover recommended preventive services without cost sharing.
  - This includes screenings for HIV, STDs, depression, and substance use.

Transgender Health Coverage

- The transgender population is more likely to live in poverty and less likely to have health insurance than the general population.
  - In one survey of transgender individuals, nearly half (48%) of respondents postponed or went without care when they were sick because they could not afford it (Kates et al., 2018).
- Many health plans include transgender-specific exclusions that deny transgender individuals' coverage of services that they provide people who are not transgender.
  - Such as mental health services and hormone therapy.

HEALTHY PEOPLE 2020 AND HEALTHY PEOPLE 2030

Healthy People 2020 included a new topic area for "Lesbian, Gay, Bisexual, and Transgender Health." This was the first time for our federal government to have LGBT in the Healthy People program.

Healthy People 2020 focused heavily on social determinants of health, such as oppression and discrimination. The objectives for LGBT health in healthy people 2020 focused heavily on "population-based data systems" and surveys that identified LGBT people. In Healthy People 2030, the focus is still on the collection of data on LGBT health issues with a new emphasis on improving the health of LGBTQ adolescents in particular:

> Collecting population-level data is key to meeting the needs of LGBT people, but not all state and national surveys include questions about sexual orientation and gender identity. Adding these types of questions to surveys can help inform effective health promotion strategies for LGBT people.
>
> LGBT adolescents are especially at risk for being bullied, thinking about and dying from suicide, and using illegal drugs. School- and family-based interventions can help reduce these behaviors and improve health in LGBT adolescents. (Office of Disease Prevention and Health Promotion, n.d.)

Nursing Considerations for LGBTQ Health and Legal Rights

LGBTQ rights have expanded in the 21st century. Several landmark rulings by the Supreme Court have extended fundamental rights to LGBTQ people living in the country. It is vital for nurses and other healthcare providers to understand the local, state, and federal laws surrounding LGBTQ people. This knowledge can equip the nurse to provide LGBTQ people with culturally competent care and better understand the health disparities. For instance, someone living in a state that does not extend discrimination protections to LGBTQ people might be hesitant to disclose their sexuality to nurses and healthcare providers out of fear that they might lose their insurance or housing if they are outed to the wrong person.

Fast Facts

Laws protecting LGBTQ people from discrimination differ at the local, state, and federal levels. In many states, LGBTQ people can be evicted and be refused services.

Chapter 17 Advocacy, Policy, and Legal Issues for LGBTQ Populations

Laws and policies are intrinsically linked to our acceptance of LGBTQ people and, ultimately, their health and well-being. Nurses must advocate for LGBTQ rights and protections in every domain, and one way to do that is to support antidiscrimination protections for LGBTQ people. At the time of publication of this book, the House of Representatives introduced and passed the Equality Act. The Equality Act would provide consistent and explicit antidiscrimination protections for LGBTQ people across key areas of life, including employment, housing, credit, education, public spaces and services, federally funded programs, and jury service.

Nurses may wonder how advocating for policies and laws for LGBTQ people is important to nursing and healthcare. Research from the John Hopkins University showed that suicide attempts among LGBTQ adolescents by 14% following the Supreme Court ruling in 2015 made same-sex marriage the law of the land. This type of judgment showed our youth that they are loved and accepted in our country and can legally love someone regardless of their sexual orientation and gender identity. The humanizing power in these types of policy changes can significantly impact the mental and physical well-being of LGBTQ people in our country. As the nation's largest healthcare profession, nurses are pivotal in advocating for policies that will improve the lives of LGBTQ people.

Fast Facts

Advocating for legislation and policies to protect LGBTQ people from discrimination is important to improving the health and well-being of LGBTQ people in our country. LGBTQ adolescent suicide dropped by 14% after the legalization of same-sex marriage.

Further Reading

Cahill, S. R. (2018). Legal and policy issues for LGBT patients with cancer or at elevated risk of cancer. *Seminars in Oncology Nursing, 34*(1), 90–98. https://doi.org/10.1016/j.soncn.2017.12.006

Family Caregiver Alliance. (n.d.). *Legal issues for LGBT caregivers.* Retrieved February 15, 2021, from https://www.caregiver.org/resource/legal-issues-lgbt-caregivers/

Kates, J., Ranji, U., Beamesderfer, A., Salganicoff, A., & Dawson, L. (2018, May). *Health and access to care and coverage for lesbian, gay, bisexual, and transgender individuals in the U.S.* http://files.kff.org/attachment/Issue-Brief-Health-and-Access-to-Care-and-Coverage-for-LGBT-Individuals-in-the-US

Mayo-Adam, E. (2020, January 30). *LGBTQ family law and policy in the United States.* Oxford Research Encyclopedia of Politics. https://oxfordre.com/politics/view/10.1093/acrefore/9780190228637.001.0001/acrefore-9780190228637-e-1216

Office of Disease Prevention and Health Promotion. (n.d.). *LGBT.* Healthy People 2030. U.S. Department of Health and Human Services. Retrieved February 15, 2021, from https://health.gov/healthypeople/objectives-and-data/browse-objectives/lgbt

Simmons-Duffin, S. (2020, June 12). *Transgender health Protections reversed By Trump administration.* https://www.npr.org/sections/health-shots/2020/06/12/868073068/transgender-health-protections-reversed-by-trump-administration

Wang, T., Kelman, E., & Cahill, S. (2016, September). *What the new affordable care act nondiscrimination rule means for providers and LGBT patients.* https://fenwayhealth.org/wp-content/uploads/HHS-ACA-1557-LGBT-Non-Discimination-Brief.pdf

Williams Institute. (2020, July 29). *How many same-sex couples in the us are raising children?* https://williamsinstitute.law.ucla.edu/publications/same-sex-parents-us/

18

Healthcare Equality Index

The Healthcare Equality Index (HEI) is a benchmarking tool from the Human Rights Campaign (HRC) that examines healthcare organizations' commitment to equity and inclusion of LGBT patients, visitors, and their employees. This chapter explores the background and significance of the HEI and how nurses can spearhead designation at their institutions.

In this chapter, you will learn:

1. About the HEI
2. How the HEI is shaping healthcare to become more LGBTQ inclusive
3. The importance of your organization obtaining HEI designation and what that means to LGBTQ patients and nurses

HUMAN RIGHTS CAMPAIGN AND THE HEALTHCARE EQUALITY INDEX

The HRC was founded in 1980 and is considered one of the first political action committees for LGBTQ people. The HRC is the largest LGBTQ civil rights organization in the United States. Resources provided by the HRC encompass marriage, adoption, schooling, and other aspects of human life.

The HEI was first introduced in 2007 and helped set the LGBTQ-inclusive care standard in America. The HEI is used to gauge how well healthcare organizations provide quality care and create a quality work environment for LGBTQ people. The key areas that are evaluated by the HEI:

1. Nondiscrimination and staffing training
2. Patient services and support
3. Employee benefits and policies
4. Patient and community engagement

The HEI is an essential metric. It has driven hospitals and health centers across the country to demonstrate their concern and engage in better efforts to improve LGBTQ equity within their institutions. The HEI is primarily for inpatient facilities that provide medical and surgical care. Specialty hospitals and individual outpatient healthcare facilities may participate by request.

Fast Facts

The HEI is a tool used to recognize high-performing hospitals and healthcare institutions that demonstrate equitable treatment and inclusion of LGBTQ patients and staff.

Human Rights Campaign by the Numbers

- Over 150,000 hours of training in LGBTQ patient-centered care was provided to staff at participating facilities.
- In 2020, a record 765 healthcare facilities actively participated in the HEI 2020 survey—that number was up from 122 in 2012.

Fast Facts

A total of 765 hospitals across the United States participated in the HEI in 2020.

Human Rights Campaign Scoring

Hospitals and healthcare institutions are scored based on how many LGBT-inclusive policies and practices that are in place. Each of the four scoring areas has different metrics for organizations to meet and are based on the following criteria:

- Nondiscrimination and staff training (40 points)
  - Patient nondiscrimination
  - Equal visitation
  - Employment nondiscrimination
  - Staff training
- Patient services and support (30 points)
  - LGBTQ patient services and support
  - Transgender patient services and support
  - Patient self-identification
  - Medical decision-making
- Employee benefits and policies (20 points)
  - Equal benefits
  - Additional support for LGBTQ employees
  - Healthcare benefits impacting transgender employees
- Patient and community engagement (10 points)
  - LGBTQ community engagement and marketing
  - Understand the needs of LGBTQ patients and communities

Top Performers and Leaders in LGBTQ Healthcare

- Scores from 80 to 95 (out of 100) are rated as a Top Performer designation. This implies that facilities are going above and beyond the basics of LGBTQ care.
  - In 2020, 193 facilities earned this designation.
- To achieve a score of 100 points and earn the designation as a Leader in LGBTQ Healthcare Equality, organizations must also include transgender-inclusive healthcare benefits to their employees.
  - In 2020, 495 healthcare facilities met this standard.

Fast Facts

Hospitals designated as a Top Leader on the HEI have significantly higher overall ratings of patient experience scores than non-HEI Leader hospitals.

Hospitals and healthcare centers compete for patients, nurses, and employees. In turn, these same groups also seek out information about the hospital where they seek care or employment. The HEI can help hospitals improve the patient experience through a more informed understanding of the LGBTQ community.

Research has found a positive statistically significant relationship between HEI Leader designation and patients rating a "9" or "10" (10-point scale) on Hospital Consumer Assessment of Healthcare Providers and Systems (HCAHPS) survey relating to the hospital's overall rating (0 = worst, 10 = best; DiLeo et al., 2020). Compared to hospitals that participate in the HEI, nonparticipating hospitals are 33% less likely to have nondiscrimination policies that include sexual orientation and gender identity. They are 37% less likely to have an LGBTQ-inclusive employment nondiscrimination policy (HRC, 2020a, 2020b).

HRC's HEI is an essential benchmarking tool in LGBTQ healthcare equality. The HEI catalyzes organizations to embark on a journey to improve the provisions of care and employment for LGBTQ people and distinguish excellence in LGBTQ healthcare equality. Nurses working or seeking employment at these organizations can take pride in the quality of care that is being delivered to LGBTQ patients and to the many employees who identify as LGBTQ.

Fast Facts

The HEI assures that the healthcare facility has the information and resources needed to ensure that LGBTQ patients can access patient-centered and culturally competent care.

Further Reading

DiLeo, R., Borkowski, N., O'Connor, S. J., Datti, P., & Weech-Maldonado, R. (2020). The relationship between "leader in LGBT healthcare equality" designation and hospitals' patient experience scores. *Journal of Healthcare Management, 65*(5), 366–377. https://doi.org/10.1097/jhm-d-19-00177

Human Rights Campaign. (2020a). *HEI scoring criteria.* https://www.thehrc foundation.org/professional-resources/hei-scoring-criteria

Human Rights Campaign. (2020b). *Healthcare equality index 2020.* https:// www.hrc.org/resources/healthcare-equality-index

19

Developing and Integrating LGBTQ Content Into Nursing Education

Education and lifelong learning are at the heart of nursing. When nurses are taught well, education can impact the knowledge, attitudes, and skills of learners. Education is the key to help nurses develop LGBTQ cultural competency, improve the overall care for LGBTQ patients, and lastly, improve general health equity for LGBTQ people. This chapter will explore how nurses can integrate and develop LGBTQ curriculum or learnings into their programs and institutions.

In this chapter, you will learn:

1. The role of nursing education in addressing LGBTQ health disparities
2. Recommendations for incorporating LGBTQ health content into nursing curriculums, programs, and educational offerings
3. How to develop LGBTQ-focused cultural competency training

HETERONORMATIVE NURSING CURRICULA

Nursing programs across the country have begun to include content about LGBTQ health. However, gaps continue to exist regarding the placement and prioritization of content in an already rigorous and rigid curriculum. Recent research has suggested that nursing programs do not provide students with a consistent or systematic curriculum specific to LGBTQ health. In some reports, nursing faculty spend only 2 to 3 hours of instruction time on LGBTQ health, including theory, skills labs, and clinical practice environments. Perhaps the most significant barrier to incorporating LGBTQ content into the nursing curriculum is that the pedagogical framework used to inform nursing students is largely heteronormative (Englund et al., 2019). Heteronormativity, by definition, is the incorrect assumption that all persons are heterosexual by default (Smith & Fitzwater, 2017).

An examination of nursing health textbooks found that LGBTQ content was lacking meaningful substance. Nursing texts describe the LGBTQ population in general teams and fail to define LGBTQ terminology and vocabulary. Another area that falls short in nursing education is the primary focus on STDs and HIV as the main discussion points (de Guzman et al., 2018). While this is a health risk for LGBTQ people, the focus on this one risk behavior in nursing texts diminished the population's health disparities by ignoring their other health risks.

With this lack of knowledge, nursing students are ill-equipped to provide culturally competent care to LGBTQ people. Research has shown that upwards of 80% of practicing nurses have had no education or training in caring for LGBTQ people. Approximately 30% of nurses reported feeling uncomfortable or unsure of their comfort level regarding caring for LGBTQ patients (Englund et al., 2019). As the nurses represent the largest workforce, we can impact the health outcomes for LGBTQ people, but we cannot do that without the necessary knowledge and competencies.

Teaching nurses and nursing students about LGBTQ health and caring for LGBTQ people is the first step in improving their knowledge. With that knowledge, attitudes about LGBTQ people can be enhanced when students have the opportunity to engage in face-to-face encounters with LGBTQ people. Research with medical and nursing students has shown that increased encounters and knowledge of LGBTQ people directly correlates to an increase in comfort level with caring for LGBTQ people and more positive attitudes (Orgel, 2017). Interactive experiences provide students with opportunities to strengthen their clinical skills and care for LGBTQ people (Orgel, 2017).

Methods for improving nursing students' attitudes toward LGBTQ people:

- Panel discussions
- Guest speakers
- Community outreach

- Interactive experiences
  - Role-playing
  - Simulation
  - Clinical assignments

TEACHING IN THE CLASSROOM AND CLINICAL SETTINGS

Classroom learning is ideal for teaching a large amount of information, laying the foundation for the clinical setting and critical thinking skills (see Boxes 19.1–19.3). Didactics and lectures can be dedicated to LGBTQ health content, introducing terminology and exploring sexual orientation and gender identity concepts. Many resources are available to those constructing learnings to use as starting points, such as chapters from textbooks, existing presentations (such as the National LGBTQ Health Education), and local organizations. Culturally competent care of LGBTQ people can also be interwoven throughout the curriculum when discussing other vital concepts and exemplars.

Exhibit 19.1 shows some examples of case studies that could be used in a concept-based curriculum. These studies highlight how LGBTQ health can have a place throughout the program.

Exhibit 19.1

Example Case Studies for a Nursing Curriculum

- Concepts: Coping, communication, and patient-centered care
  - Exemplars: Anxiety, stress, substance misuse, and therapeutic communication.
  - Michelle is a transgender patient who presents to the ED because of a panic attack while at work. During the assessment, Michelle tells the nurse that she takes the occasional Ativan from a friend and usually has a "few" drinks every night. Michelle says that the stress of her job, her transition, and being overwhelmed with life is just too much at times.
  - Additional discussion for this case can explore the social determinants of health and health disparities within the LGBTQ population.

- Concepts: Immunity, patient-centered care, and ethical and legal practice and sexuality
  - Exemplars: Informed consent, therapeutic communication, health promotion, and vaccines, STDs.
  - Max is a 17-year-old male who visits a community health clinic. Max is worried that he might have an STD. The nurse can tell that Max is extremely anxious and embarrassed. Max states that this is the first scare and is very nervous. He does not want his parents to find out that he has

been having sex with men and is worried about what would happen at home and school if people found out.

■ Routine vaccinations such as HPV can be discussed. Barriers to care can be examined, health promotion in the LGBTQ community, and the nurse's role. Legal implications for nurses can also be explored, such as informed consent and the age of consent in the state.

BOX 19.1 RECOMMENDATIONS FOR FACULTY

- Evaluate the current curriculum and conduct a gap analysis.
- Develop confidence and competence in teaching LGBTQ content.
  - Partner with local and national LGBTQ organizations.
  - Seminars, workshops, faculty development symposiums, and web-based training.

BOX 19.2 RECOMMENDATIONS FOR PRELICENSURE CURRICULUMS

- Evaluate the current curriculum and conduct a gap analysis.
- Foster open dialogue in the classroom to discuss the topic.
- Address specific health concerns for LGBTQ people and address misconceptions.
- Allow for specific clinical rotations that will allow exposure to LGBTQ people.
- Include guest speakers and/or panel discussions on LGBTQ health issues and concerns.
- Teach and validate effective communication strategies.
- Use case studies and simulations that include LGBTQ people.
- Discuss resources for LGBTQ people with students.
- Conduct a seminar or reflective assignment/discussion on the unconscious and conscious biases.
- Ground activities in the concept of social justice and the development of cultural competence.

BOX 19.3 RECOMMENDATIONS FOR GRADUATE EDUCATION

- Evaluate the current curriculum and conduct a gap analysis.
- Have specific classes or content related to caring for LGBTQ people and other vulnerable populations.
  - Ensure that transgender people receive dedicated content.
- Incorporate content that addresses specific health concerns, risk factors, and health promotion for the LGBTQ population.
- Include guest speakers and panel discussions with LGBTQ individuals who have had experience with healthcare and providers.
- Teach effective communication strategies to engage with LGBTQ people and foster a safe and inclusive environment.
- Incorporate evidence-based practice and research on LGBTQ health and care into courses and assignments.
- Inform students of resources that are available to LGBTQ people and for advanced nursing practice.
- Utilize clinical simulations with standardized patients using trained actors to portray LGBTQ people.

CONTINUING PROFESSIONAL EDUCATION

As a profession, nurses are expected to continually update their knowledge, skill, and behaviors of their clinical practice setting and licensure requirements. Many national nursing organizations, such as the American Nurses Association, support the fundamental importance of lifelong learning and professional competence. Continuing education (CE) for professional nurses can be delivered in many formats to meet the various needs of nurses. Organizations can conduct grand rounds, offer webinars or asynchronous learning, journal clubs and conferences. It is critical that educators and nurse planners planning educational events, such as conferences, ensure that LGBTQ-specific content is included in non-LGBTQ-specific learning opportunities.

Several organizations, such as the Human Rights Campaign (HRC) and the National LGBTQIA+ Health Education Center, offer free CE credits to healthcare professionals. Practicing nurses may find these educational offerings useful for clinical practice and knowledge. Nursing professional development specialists and nurse educators may also find their resources helpful to use as a sounding board and guide for developing education that fits their organization's needs.

DEVELOPING LGBTQ CULTURAL COMPETENCY EDUCATION

- Cultural competency education is becoming a key component in healthcare education and professional development.
  - The term has been used interchangeably with diversity education, cultural sensitivity training, and multicultural workshops.
- Cultural competency is commonly understood as a set of congruent behaviors, knowledge, attitudes, and policies that enable practical work in cross-cultural situations.
  - Cultural competency training aims to increase knowledge and skills to improve one's ability to interact with different cultural groups effectively.
- LGBTQ cultural competency training has been developed and implemented to improve healthcare and social service delivery to LGBTQ patients and clients.
- Education components will need to be updated regularly to reflect current health policies, laws, research, LGBTQ statistics, and recommendation.

Adult Learning Theory

A critical theory to help guide educational design for practicing nurses is the Adult Learning Theory.

- Adult learners are not like younger students who are used to learning information to take a test.
- Adults are often internally motivated.
- Adults enter the room with a strong sense of self, knowledge, and are firmly attached to their beliefs, ethics, and style.
- Adult learners will often be resistant to information that is being imposed on them.
  - For LGBTQ cultural competence, it is essential to understand where the nurses are coming from and how this content will impact their care.
  - Nurses want to learn things that will have an immediate impact or relevance to their nursing role.
  - To teach adult learners, include examples that apply to the patients they care for in the organization and practice setting and how it relates to the hospital's overall mission and policies.

Nursing faculty and educators have a responsibility to prepare their graduates and practicing nurses to meet the diverse healthcare of the LGBTQ community. LGBTQ content must be incorporated throughout the nursing curriculums and programs. Research has proven that nurses are more confident in their clinical skills if they know and encounter people who identify as LGBTQ. Nursing programs have lagged behind other healthcare professions in incorporating LGBTQ content and let this chapter be a call to action for all nurses. Education is at the heart of nursing and is essential to ensure that LGBTQ patients receive the culturally competent care they deserve.

Fast Facts

Upward of 80% of practicing nurses have had no education or training in caring for LGBTQ people. Approximately 30% of nurses reported feeling uncomfortable or unsure of their comfort level regarding caring for LGBTQ patients.

Interactive experiences such as role-playing, simulation, and clinical assignments provide students with opportunities to improve their clinical skills and care for LGBTQ people.

Increased encounters and knowledge of LGBTQ people increase both the nurse's attitude and comfort level regarding LGBTQ people.

Further Reading

American Nurses Association. (2018). *Nursing advocacy for LGBTQ+ populations.* https://www.nursingworld.org/~49866e/globalassets/practiceand policy/ethics/nursing-advocacy-for-lgbtq-populations.pdf

Caboral-Stevens, M., Rosario-Sim, M., & Lovence, K. (2018). Cultural competence of NURSING Faculty of the LGBT Population. *Nursing and Primary Care, 2*(3), 1–4. https://doi.org/10.33425/2639-9474.1063

De Guzman, F. L., Moukoulou, L. N., Scott, L. D., & Zerwic, J. J. (2018). LGBT inclusivity in health assessment textbooks. *Journal of Professional Nursing, 34*(6), 483–487. https://doi.org/10.1016/j.profnurs.2018.03.001

Englund, H., Basler, J., & Meine, K. (2019). Using simulation to improve students' proficiency in taking the sexual history of patients identifying as LGBTQ: A pilot study. *Clinical Simulation in Nursing, 37*, 1–4. https://doi.org/10.1016/j.ecns.2019.07.007

Kroning, M. (2018). Lesbian, gay, bisexual, and transgender education in nursing. *Nurse Educator, 43*(1), 41. https://doi.org/10.1097/nne.00000 00000000429

Orgel, H. (2017). Improving LGBT cultural competence in nursing students: An integrative review. *The ABNF Journal, 28*(1), 14–18.

Smith, P., & Fitzwater, J. (2017). Incorporating lesbian, gay, bisexual, and transgender (LGBT) health concepts into nursing curricula: What nursing faculty should know. *Faculty Presentations.* Presentation. Submission 2. https://digitalcommons.linfield.edu/nursfac_pres/2

Appendix: Professional Organizations and Resources for Nurses

This section contains various resources for the nurse to learn more information about LGBTQ health and various resources for LGBTQ patients.

The Trevor Project (www.trevorproject.org). The Trevor Project provides suicide prevention efforts for the LGBTQ+ community. The organization features a hotline that connects callers in need with trained counselors and other important resources.

LGBT National Hotline (www.glbthotline.org). The LGBT National Hotline provides phone, chat, email, and text lines for different demographics within the LGBTQ+ community, including youth and senior lines. The hotline also provides resources for allies.

Trans Lifeline (www.translifeline.org). The Trans Lifeline offers emotional and financial support to trans people in need or crisis. Nurses can take advantage of many helpful resources, including a mailing list.

GLMA (www.glma.org). The Gay and Lesbian Medical Association offers a useful directory of healthcare professionals who provide trustworthy care to the LGBTQ+ community. Nurses and patients alike can use the searchable directory to locate providers.

Center of Excellence for Transgender Health (https://prevention .ucsf.edu/transhealth). The Center of Excellence for Transgender Health aims to increase access to comprehensive, effective, and affirming healthcare services for transgender and gender-variant communities.

Center for American Progress (LGBT) (www.americanprogress .org/issues/lgbt). Dedicated to improving the lives of Americans through ideas and action, combining bold policy ideas with a modern communications platform to help shape the national debate. CAP is designed to provide long-term leadership and support to the progressive movement.

Fenway Community Health and Fenway Institute (www.fenway health.org). Fenway's mission is to enhance the well-being of the LGBTQ community and all people in its neighborhoods and beyond through access to the highest quality healthcare, education, research, and advocacy.

Healthy People 2020 (www.healthypeople2020.org). Produced by the Office of Disease Prevention and Health Promotion (ODPHP), this is the key science-based, 10-year national objectives for improving the health of all Americans which historically includes LGBT health. LGBTQ health experts produced an LGBT compendium document to Healthy People 2010.

LGBT Cancer (www.lgbtcancer.org). The National LGBT Cancer Project is the United States' first and leading LGBT cancer survivor support and advocacy nonprofit organization, committed to improving the health of LGBT cancer survivors with peer-to-peer support.

LGBT Health Journal (www.liebertpub.com/lgbt). Published six times per year, this journal profiles new and cutting-edge science-based LGBTQ health research articles on current and emerging issues.

The National Coalition for LGBT Health (https://healthhiv.org). The National Coalition for LGBT Health project seeks to destigmatize LGBTQ healthcare and raise awareness of LGBTQ health disparities. The coalition also seeks to expand cultural competency for the diverse LGBTQ population and to improve both access to, and utilization of, healthcare resources. PFLAG National is a member organization.

National HIV/AIDS Strategy (www.hiv.gov). Launched in 2009, The White House issued the NHAS for the United States to reflect many of the approaches the CDC believes will reduce HIV incidence.

The World Professional Association for Transgender Health, Inc (WPATH) (www.wpath.org). Interdisciplinary professional and educational organization devoted to transgender health. Its stated mission is to promote evidence-based care, education, research, advocacy, public policy, and respect in transgender health. To support that mission, the organization engages in clinical and academic research to improve the quality of care provided to transsexual, transgender, and gender-expansive individuals globally.

Lambda Legal (www.lambdalegal.org). A national organization committed to achieving full recognition of the civil rights of LGBT people and everyone living with HIV through impact litigation, education, and public policy work.

The Joint Commission (www.jointcomission.org). Advancing Effective Communication, Cultural Competence, and Patient- and Family-Centered Care for the Lesbian, Gay, Bisexual, and Transgender (LGBT) Community: How to advance effective communication, cultural competence, and patient- and family-centered care specifically for the LGBT community.

Human Rights Campaign–Healthy Equality Index (https://www .hrc.org/resources/healthcare-equality-index). Promoting equitable and inclusive care for LGBTQ patients and their families.

National LGBTQIA+ Health Education Center (https://www .lgbtqiahealtheducation.org). Provides educational programs, resources, and consultation to healthcare organizations with the goal of optimizing quality, cost-effective healthcare for lesbian, gay, bisexual, transgender, queer, intersex, asexual, and all sexual and gender minority (LGBTQIA+) people.

Health and Human Services: LGBT (https://www.hhs.gov/programs/ topic-sites/lgbt/index.html). HHS works to ensure that LGBT Americans, families, and communities receive equal access to health services by providing enhanced resources for LGBT health issues; developing better information regarding LGBT health needs; and working to close the LGBT health disparity gap that currently exists.

National Resource Center on LGBT Aging (https://www.lgbtaging center.org). The country's first and only technical assistance resource center aimed at improving the quality of services and supports offered to LGBT older adults.

Index

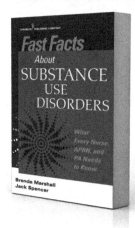
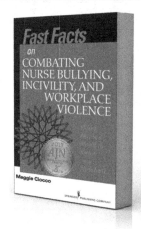
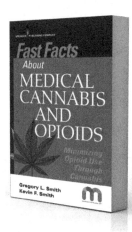
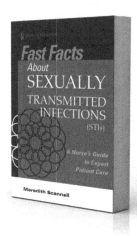

Printed in the United States
by Baker & Taylor Publisher Services